The Caregiver's Companion

OTHER BOOKS BY PATRICIA JEAN SMITH

The Golf Widow's Revenge (1986)
Double Bind (1991)
A Song For My Daughter (2008)

The Caregiver's Companion

Patricia Jean Smith

Rock's Mills Press
Oakville, Ontario
2022

Rock's Mills Press
www.rocksmillspress.com

The author and publisher gratefully acknowledge permission from the following to include material under copyright in this book:

Gary Geddes, "Riding the Wild Horse, Memory: A Review," first published in the *Vancouver Sun*, September 2016.

Dr. Helen Kennerly and Dr. Udo Kischka, *Surviving Stroke: The Story of a Neurologist and His Family*, published by Robinson of the Little, Brown Book Group, May 2020.

Thomas King, *The Inconvenient Indian: A Curious Account of Native People in North America*, Anchor Canada, a division of Random House of Canada Limited, August 2013.

Alberto Rios, his poem, "When Giving is All We Have."

Ron Smith, *The Defiant Mind: Living Inside a Stroke*, Ronsdale Press, August 2016.

David Travland Ph.D & Rhonda Travland, *The Tough and Tender Caregiver: A Handbook for the Well Spouse*, April 2009.

Jon Turk, *Crocodiles and Ice: A Journey into Deep Wild*, Oolichan Books, September 2016.

For information about this book, please contact the publisher at
customer.service@rocksmillspress.com
or visit us online at www.rocksmillspress.com.

for Ron,

Flora, Lochlan and Anja

The burden that is well borne becomes light.
—Ovid

Contents

Preface / xi

Part Three: Mind and Matter/Body and Soul

Preface

On November 19, 2012 my husband, Ron Smith, suffered a massive ischemic stroke to his brain stem. During his recovery, still an ongoing process, he wrote a powerful book about his experience—*The Defiant Mind: Living Inside a Stroke*. Having lost the use of his right side, including his arm and hand, he composed the work with his left index finger, typing the work's three hundred plus pages one letter at a time. Today we both continue to cope with the disabling aftershocks of his stroke.

Since the book's publication Ron has spoken to literally thousands of people—fellow stroke survivors, health care professionals, writing groups, arts gatherings, diverse clubs, library goers and general readers. During these events I was often asked if I had written my side of the story. My response to this question was usually a wan smile and a shrug. To be honest, writing such a book was not something I felt capable of doing. Being a caregiver 24/7, and maintaining a large house and garden, sapped most of my energy. When there was free time in which to write, I preferred recreation and escape. Writing a book about caregiving was not where my literary aspirations lay. I had other projects. Nothing to do with stroke. Or with caregiving.

Such was my state of mind until Thursday morning, September 20, 2018. Ron had agreed to speak at a book club hosted by our neighbour and friend, Bev Coolican.

Inevitably, late in the meeting, over coffee and pastries, the familiar questions came up.

"What was it like for you, Pat? Where's your book? Where's the companion volume?"

I gave the ladies my wan smile, my wry shrug.

"But you must write it!" they insisted. "And we'll help! We've had experience assisting an author produce a book."

Appreciative of their fulsome praise for *The Defiant Mind*, I was taken aback by their enthusiasm for a potential book of mine. Their excitement was contagious.

Yes, I thought.

Why not?

One way or another, I'd been a caregiver for many years, intensely so during the first three years, after Ron had left the hospital and continued to recuperate at home. My experience might be worth sharing. My voice might be helpful. With the sale of our large home and the move into our townhouse, my workload had lessened. I now had more time to write, I realized. And, if I needed help, I'd have these discerning ladies to talk with. But most importantly, for the first time since Ron's stroke, I also felt I had the emotional and physical strength to accept the challenge the book club and so many others had posed.

I knew already the kind of book I wanted to write. It would not be a training manual with instructions for dressing, bathing, tripping hazards and so forth; nor an hour-by-hour guide to cooking meals and managing time; nor an analysis of care homes, their virtues and their limitations—valuable as these instructional books would be. I wanted my book—this book—to be something else: a companion, in the sense of a compassionate ally, for those who find themselves, perhaps abruptly, needing to care for others. I would begin with what Ron's stroke meant to me as well as to him and write about the critical demands and the marvellous rewards of caring—of exercising and extending care. I would also write about the adventures that otherwise would not have chanced our way had it not been for Ron's stroke.

Strokes wreak havoc on marriages. Less than half survive a brain attack. Caring for stroke survivors or other physically and mentally challenged family members is exhausting work. Every part of one's being is tested. And, once a caregiver has managed to achieve a state of balance in her (or his) life, revisiting the past—the shock, the trials, the grief—and putting it down in writing is not a prospect that appeals.

Yet, over time, I have come to appreciate that being a caregiver is essential for anyone who wants to live a meaningful and satisfying life. If we were to honour the values that caregiving embodies, we would all become nurturers of life and of the marvellous Earth we are privileged to call home. We would proudly call ourselves caregivers.

By sharing the wisdom I have gleaned from my experience and by sharing the example of other caregivers, stroke survivors, medical practitioners, friends, family, and the support I have found in books, I trust that I might help ease the burden a caregiver daily assumes; that I might offer a compassionate voice in times of despair and suggest some tips for the road ahead. I want to be a companion and a friend who advocates for caregivers everywhere, who illustrates the true value of this work, and who demonstrates that caregiving is the most vital thing we do.

Patricia Jean Smith
Nanoose Bay, BC
May 2021

The Caregiver's Companion

PART ONE
The Brain Attack

CHAPTER ONE
Life Goes Sideways

I was sixty-five the day my life changed, the day it went sideways. My husband, Ron, and I were living in our retirement dream home. It had a timber frame super-structure resting on concrete Arxx block walls rising to the gables and was topped by a metal roof. The appraiser our insurance company had hired said the house should be proof against natural disasters such as fire, flood and earthquake. Like the Pantheon, ours was a building that would last.

Ron and I had designed and built our new home with the help of his brother, Brian. We all thought it beautiful, nestled as it was, when finished, into a woodland of fir, cedar, hemlock, arbutus, holly, maple and alder on a half acre overlooking two ponds, a fountain, two fairways and the waterway which meandered through Fairwinds golf course. We were mere steps from the clubhouse and the first tee.

One of the unique features of our house design was that it included two main floor studies—one for *him*, large enough to house his entire library, and a smaller one for *her*—a room of my own, one of Virginia Woolf's requirements for women who wish to write—with a large balcony where I could sunbathe, just off the kitchen.

With Brian for back up, Ron and I had boldly taken on the challenge of registering as the official Owner/

Builder. We had applied for the building permit and appeared before the Board of Variance, obtaining two variances for the price of one. We had been our own contractor and had hired all the workers—the surveyor, the excavator, the engineer and our site supervisor. We had opened accounts at building supply stores; we had scouted out plumbers, electricians, cement finishers, drywallers, and painters. We had sourced door makers, window makers, skylight fabricators and sawmills for the external cedar shakes. We had picked out cabinets and countertops, appliances, door hardware, toilets and faucets; chosen landscapers and stone masons.

We had solved problems.

When we ultimately moved into our custom-built home, we could recite the history of every nook and cranny. Having put all our resources, labour and imagination into house building, we turned our attention to the goal of our endeavours—the provision of an environmentally sensitive, creative space in which to work and to play. Not that work and play are mutually exclusive. In truth they can be one. Every artist, artisan, athlete and child knows that.

On the day in question, Monday, November 19, 2012, the day of the stroke, I was just about to leave for my end of season luncheon with my golfing group. The lunch was an annual outing we all looked forward to— our conversation being infinitely superior to our golf. And what woman doesn't look forward to enjoying a meal that she hasn't had to cook?

While I was getting dressed to go out Ron came into the bedroom and announced that he wasn't feeling well.

"Should I stay home?" I asked, my concern for his well-being mitigated by my disappointment at the prospect of having to miss my outing.

"No. No. Go ahead. I might be getting the flu. Nothing to worry about. I think I'll take a nap."

Reassured, I left for lunch. When I returned home later in the afternoon, I found Ron still in bed, still feeling *odd*.

"Perhaps we should head to the hospital," I suggested.

"Good God. No."

It was later, around dinnertime, after much nagging on my part and continuing refusal on his, before I finally convinced Ron to get checked out. *He must be feeling terrible*, I thought, as I backed the car out of the garage, and we drove to the Emergency Department of the Nanaimo Regional General Hospital. After sitting for three hours in the waiting room, Ron finally got to see a doctor, a doctor who convinced him that he should stay in the hospital for five days for observation.

No small feat, I thought upon hearing the news. Ron, like many men, is very reluctant to go to hospital, let alone stay in one. He would rather man up and tough it out at home.

After making this major decision we returned to the waiting room while preparations were made for his admission to the hospital. We were still sitting in the Emergency waiting room when Ron turned to me and said in a barely audible whisper, "Run and get help. I'm dying." Then he slid off his chair onto the floor.

Throughout my adult life I have attempted to remain calm in a crisis. Perhaps this attitude has carried over from the Royal Canadian Lifesaving training I received in my youth.

Row, throw, tow, go.

Only as a last resort should a lifeguard jump into the water to attempt to save a drowning person. Stay calm and do not jeopardize your own life in a rescue if possible.

Yet, when your husband of forty-four years whispers that he is dying, you instantly leap from your chair, race across the waiting room to the nearest doctor's station, shrieking, "Help, help, my husband's dying." My pandemonium triggered immediate results. Orderlies and nurses materialized and hoisted Ron onto a stretcher. As I scrambled to stay out of the way, they rushed Ron into one of the rooms in Emergency and hooked him up to monitors and IV drips.

I was numb.

I could tell from the conversations I was overhearing that the response I was observing was deadly serious. Everyone was calm, efficient, even chatty in a soothing way, but unmistakably intense. And incredibly methodical. Precise.

Once Ron's condition had stabilized, and he had been dressed in a hospital gown and tagged with a plastic ID bracelet, peace and quiet returned. The lights in Emergency dimmed, and after more sitting and waiting, I decided to go home.

It was 2:30 a.m.

When I returned to the hospital at mid-morning the next day, I heard Ron was scheduled to be moved to a room in the Acute Care Ward on the Fourth Floor. I was told by a nurse that the consensus of medical opinion was that he had suffered a stroke, although nothing definite had yet showed up on his CT scan.

Knowing nothing about strokes and their possible devastating effects, I tried to remain calm. Ron's mental faculties seemed intact, but his physical powers were worsening. His voice was garbled, and he was losing movement on the right side of his body. I had brought his housecoat, slippers and some toiletries with me. When the time for the move to the Acute Ward came, I gathered up his things and dutifully followed the lady who pushed his stretcher from the recently opened, state-of-the-art Emergency quarters, into an elevator located in the heart of the original hospital building. When we reached the Fourth Floor, she manoeuvred him down a narrow passage through a crowded hall. I was shocked by the number of nurses and doctors working at temporary computer stations outside the patients' rooms; by the sight of patients, clad only in nightgowns, attached to portable IV units, slowly wending their way through the congestion, past cleaners pushing trolleys piled high with mops, buckets, cleaning supplies and bedding. The number of people coming and going was overwhelming, like a crowd in a busy, outdoor market.

Ron's bearer deftly worked her way through this throng and turned into the last room on the right at the end of the hall where she and a nurse transferred Ron to the bed by the window. I was relieved to get to the window where I took deep gulps of the outside air which flowed into the room through leaky window seals. There was one other patient in the darkened room, but it was impossible to get a glimpse of him. His bed was surrounded by white curtains. Soon he was moved out by a couple of orderlies, ostensibly for more tests. Subsequently I learned he had died.

Later I would read in Robert McCrum's *My Year Off: Rediscovering Life after a Stroke* that he felt most stroke victims were shunted to the furthermost corner of the hospital, ostensibly to be 'out of sight, out of mind.' Then as now, strokes are still a mystery.

Throughout the day various nurses and technicians came and went, checking Ron's vital signs and taking blood samples. I cannot remember if a doctor stopped by. For me, the good news was that Ron was *alive*. We could worry about the *well* later. After a long day at the hospital, I left at dusk, driving home through the November rain, to an empty house, to a cold supper for one, and a list of family and friends to email.

November 20, 2012:

> I'm sorry to report that Ron has suffered a stroke and is in hospital. He's getting excellent care and we trust he will make a complete recovery. However, he will have to stay in the hospital until he is well enough to come home. Nicole is going to come over tomorrow and that will cheer her Dad up. In the meantime, he will not be responding to his emails. I can't even tell if his laptop is on or off.
>
> Love, Pat

"*Whoa*," I say, as I reread this email. In hindsight I need to correct some of the information that I initially included in it. First and foremost, I had no idea what a stroke was. I don't think I even knew that the affected area was Ron's brain, let alone what part of it had taken the greatest hit or what the effects of this would be on his physical and emotional being. I had no idea that stroke is the number one cause of permanent disability worldwide nor that my faith in Ron's 'full recovery' would ultimately prove naïve.

As Ron and I continue to learn from other stroke survivors and their caregivers, people are woefully ignorant of stroke. People who are having strokes commonly mistake the condition for something else. Even medical people specializing in the stroke field can misdiagnose their own stroke symptoms. They conclude they are suffering from the flu, or a headache, or simply coming down with a cold. They often *go to bed*!?! When Canada's Chief Medical officer suffered his *second* stroke a few years ago, he assumed he had the flu, and *went to bed*. Recently a neurologist working in Oxford, England, and on faculty in that venerable old university, Dr. Udo Kischka, published an article in the British medical journal, the *Lancet*, in which he admitted to doing the same thing. While having a massive stroke he thought he had the flu and *went to bed*.

Ron wrote to Professor Kischka in response to his admission in the article that after thirty years as a consultant who had advised stroke survivors on therapy and recovery, he now realized how little he actually understood about the effects and consequences of stroke. When he uttered to his wife, Dr. Helen Kennerley, a clinical psychologist and university tutor, a few hours after his stroke, "This is a life-changing event," he had no idea just how life-changing it would be. Out of this insight came his understanding of the importance of stroke stories and how they could be of benefit in research and recovery. He realized how important 'listening' to patient stories could be to individual therapy. Listen and adapt, don't preach; every story will be different. Ron had long been an advocate of the significance of each patient's and caregiver's unique story. And of listening, no matter how bizarre the narrative.

This is one of the most disheartening aspects of stroke. Its symptoms are devilishly hard to diagnose, even for so-called experts in the field. And the longer it takes to get help, the more brain cells (two million per minute) are killed off and the seriousness of the stroke, especially its side-effects, increases profoundly.

Time is brain.

As for *excellent care*, when Ron's brain attack hit there was no dedicated stroke unit at the Nanaimo Hospital, nor was there a neurologist on staff. Ron did not get tPA, the clot-busting drug. At the time it was hospital policy not to administer it. Had we known then what we subsequently learned we probably would have been much better off if I had driven Ron to any of the other Island hospitals—Port Alberni, Comox, Campbell River, Duncan, even Victoria. At these hospitals he would have been given tPA. His clot might have been "busted" and his disabilities lessened.

Today stroke care in Nanaimo has markedly improved. There is a dedicated stroke ward at the hospital, a neurologist is on staff and tPA is administered to patients who are having an ischemic or blood-clot-induced stroke.

November 22, 2012:

Just a note to let you know that Ron seems to have plateaued (is this a word?) and is possibly starting to make some strides forward. Today he began to dictate his Declaration of Dependence and suggested he and Stephen Hawking go on a speaking tour together. Ron's speech is terribly garbled, but his mind appears okay.

He retains his wit. His right side, however, is not

responsive. More tests are scheduled. Eventually, I've been told, Ron might be a good candidate for the Rehab Ward, which is excellent news. He would have to get the OK from "the team" for that. In the meantime, Ron still must pass the swallow test so that he can get real food. The hospital is, of course, very crowded. Beds, equipment, and staff, etc. all in the very cramped hallways.

Nicole is here for a day or two. Ron was thrilled to see his daughter.

Love, Pat

Again, hindsight is instructive. In times of crisis, messages can get mixed. What is communicated to one person may not be fully understood by another. While I was under the impression that Ron's prospects were the prime factors in his potential move to the Rehab Ward, he was told that a bed had come up in Rehab and the physiatrists—also known as Physical Medicine and Rehabilitation (PM&R) physicians—in charge of his care didn't want to lose it. They needed to grab it ASAP before some other department nabbed the bed. Whatever the official reasons given, I believed then that Ron's getting a bed in Rehab was critically important for his recovery. I stuck close by his bedside, forgoing a walk to the nearby arbutus grove and back to the hospital through the old Chinese graveyard. Usually I found being in the presence of the giant, old trees calming. But, on the day in question, I wanted to be near Ron to keep track of any developments.

November 23, 2012:

Today saw Ron slightly improved over yesterday. Much has also happened. He's been OK'd to move to the Rehab unit as soon as he can be processed. If that doesn't happen tomorrow, then it probably won't happen until after the weekend.

His speech is still garbled but has improved. He "walked" from his bed to the door with the assistance of three physiotherapists holding on to his transfer belt to keep him on his feet. He passed the swallow test, is now allowed pureed food, and went for his first wheelchair promenade of the premises.

Dr. Hawkswood of the Rehab unit remarked that Ron might be said to have had a "mild stroke" but for the fact that he can't use his right side: leg, arm and hand. Therefore, the doctor would have to classify him as having had a "medium" stroke. He also said that there is a 90 per cent chance that Ron will not have another stroke during the first year, and an 80 per cent chance that he will not have another stroke in the second year. These sound like good odds to me.

More good news: Owen is going to be able to come for 2 or 3 days around Dec. 1. And my brother, Bill, is going to "slide across the strait" for a couple of days as well.

Nicole returns to Vancouver tomorrow. I started a

new paragraph here, since I'm not certain this should go in the "More good news" category.

I would say the crisis is over and the recovery has begun.

Love, Pat

In retrospect, the cheery, breezy tone of my emails surprises me given the catastrophic changes in Ron which were taking place before my eyes. Was I wilfully deluding myself? Is this what is meant by *being in denial*? I do remember making a conscious decision to remain positive and upbeat for Ron, whose spirits were flagging. Depression goes hand in hand with stroke. I felt I needed to be strong for both of us. I later learned that guilt and shame are feelings stroke patients commonly endure as well. Certainly, Ron was gut-wrenched that Nicole had to see him so helpless. After all, he was the parent, the one who his daughter had always looked up to.

What would she think of him now?

Ron's new room in Rehab was a welcome change from the crowded, smelly, distressing surroundings on the Acute Care Ward where Ron's second roommate had been a young insomniac, who was carrying over 200 pounds of fluid on his 140-pound frame. A nurse had told me that he had a serious case of ascites. Whether or not it was the volume of fluid that had built up or an infection, this young man also died. Was this the sort of room Robert McCrum envisioned hospitals reserved for stroke patients? Such speculation seemed too sinister to believe. On the other hand, I was a novice to the role of caregiving and inclined to absorb any and all information.

Although Ron now had three roommates on the Rehab Ward, none of them was going to die any time soon. Two of the gentlemen were recovering from surgeries that had removed diabetic limbs and they were being fitted with prosthetic legs. The third man, like Ron, was recovering from a stroke. The accommodation was comparatively spacious. There was ample room for staff, equipment, and visitors to be present all at the same time. By comparison with the Acute Care Ward, where peace and quiet did not exist, Ron's new situation was almost restful. Also, I was able to park for free on one of the neighbouring streets and walk the couple of blocks to Rehab, located in one of the "newer" sections of the hospital which, coincidentally, also housed the psychiatric and palliative care wards.

Despite my upbeat emails and the cheerful persona I adopted for Ron and for me, the experience took a physical toll. In the first week after Ron's stroke I lost ten pounds. Fortunately, I had already learned from past experience the importance of getting a good night's sleep no matter what. I continued to don my sleep mask at night and mould my bee's wax ear plugs into my ears.

* * * * *

FROM: Barbara Osaka

Hi Pat,

I understand why you would feel fatigued ... the worry and stress of Ron's stroke plus the daily trips to the hospital quickly add up to exhaustion. Is there anything that we could do to help you and Ron? Would you and Ron be up to having us visit on Sunday, or do you think it would be wiser to wait a bit longer? Please let us know what you would prefer.

Try to get some rest this evening Pat. Are you sleeping alright? ... We're hoping Ron continues to remain stable and starts to show signs of improvement. Tell him we're thinking of him and we send him our love. Take care of yourself, Pat.

Love and Hugs, Barb

Barbara Osaka is married to Ron's brother, Brian, our dream home architect. At the time of Ron's stroke, she was a Registered Community Health Nurse, working full-time in Home Nursing Care for the Vancouver Island Health Authority in Campbell River. She was a resource I called on often for information and support, especially initially. While Ron was in hospital, she gave me a copy of Jill Bolte Taylor's *My Stroke of Insight* to read. In her book the author advises all stroke survivors to *expect full recovery*. I took her advice to heart and the phrase became a daily mantra for me.

Expect full recovery. Expect full recovery. Expect full recovery.

Later, I learned that Taylor had suffered an hemorrhagic stroke (a bleed in her brain) and not an ischemic stroke, which Ron had suffered. Hemorrhagic strokes account for approximately thirteen percent of strokes while ischemic strokes account for eighty-seven percent. From my observations of survivors of both types, the outcomes appear to be different. It seems to me that survivors of hemorrhagic strokes often recover their physical mobility more quickly but are more likely to suffer cognitive difficulties.

One of the design features that Brian had insisted upon when he drew up the plans for our house was to include extra-wide doors, thirty-six inches wide instead of the customary thirty-four. Brian said he always designed his houses to be wheelchair accessible. Given that our house already had a level entry to the main floor, Ron and I agreed this added feature could be helpful should we ever need to sell our house. Never once did we think either of us would ever need a wheelchair, or that we would be so grateful for Brian's foresight.

Post-stroke treatment decisions, decisions which directly affect the quality of patient care, are often dictated by a person's living situation at home.

Are there stairs to climb?

Can the doors accommodate a wheelchair?
Does the survivor live alone?
Is there anyone who can care for her?
Or for him?

For two presumably well-educated retirees, Ron and I were acutely ignorant of stroke and all it entailed. Neither of us had family members who had suffered with the condition, nor did we have any friends or neighbours who had been afflicted by a *brain attack*—Ron's preferred term for *stroke*, a word he feels is deceptively gentle. *Stroke* comes nowhere near to conveying the major assault on the whole being—mentally, physically, and spiritually—that survivors endure. By this time, we had the results of the MRI and we knew Ron's stroke was more severe than first diagnosed. He'd have to work in earnest on his recovery. We didn't know that stroke is the number one cause of disability worldwide. And in those early days we didn't accept the idea that Ron had joined the ranks of the disabled. Definitely not! We had no idea of what lay ahead for us both. We did not realize that our world had gone sideways—that our lives had taken a ninety-degree turn. Instead of heading forward, to the realm of our hopes and dreams, we were now headed sideways towards an unknown destination.

CHAPTER TWO

HELP from the Red Cross

December 4, 2012:

STROKE PLAY

Yes, today Ron went golfing. Well, putting really. Apparently, there is a driver in Physio, but Ron will have to work a bit harder before being able to swing the "big" club.

The news from the "team" continues to be good. At present the plan is that Ron will be sent home this coming Friday at 3:30 p.m. on a weekend pass. If he and I can cope well Ron will be discharged from the hospital and treated in Rehab on an Outpatient basis.

Each day Ron seems to get a little stronger and able to do more. He is getting quite good with his "transfers" from his wheelchair and with the use of his walker. Tomorrow, Owen and I will head to the Red Cross to pick up a wheelchair, walker, bath chair, foot support, toilet stand, and bed bar. We will also practice getting Ron in and out of the car. However, his bed at the hospital will be waiting for him if we should feel at any point that we're not up to home care. At home he will be able to sleep much better, which is a major key for a quick recovery. So, keep your collective fingers crossed.

As far as visitors go, I would have to say that Ron seems to be the most popular patient on the ward. On the weekend we had visits with Bob, Peter, Marg & Gerry, and Barb & Garnet. Today we had another one with Ron's Mom, Fran, Barrie and Karen, Brian and Barb, and Guy and Terry. Tomorrow Kieran and Pattie are going to return to Vancouver via Nanaimo so they can wish Ron well.

Owen continues to be a gem, treating his Dad to personal grooming care, homemade smoothies and his Mom to chef-style dinners at home. Last night we went out for dinner followed by a movie, *Skyfall*, the latest Bond. It celebrates 50 years of the Broccoli Family Franchise and promises lots more Bonds to come. Bond fans like me (the lukewarm kind) have to give it a thumbs up.

Thanks again for all your love and support,
Pat (e Ronaldo)

One of the most depressing sides to life in the Rehab Unit was the sight of the many stroke survivors who received no visitors at all and who were left to recover all alone, without the support of friends and family.

I was upset. Apart from a couple of spouses, in particular a husband who followed the therapists around while they were treating his partner, from one apparatus to another, and a wife who instructed the nurses on how to apply ointment to a bandage, where were those who would have to care for all the other patients busy working on their recovery? When would they enter the picture?

Wasn't this the beginning of our time (in retrospect, possibly careers) as caregivers?

Everyone who has had a stroke knows how essential support and encouragement is to recovery. How these lonely people eventually made out, I have no clue, only pessimistic suspicions.

December 6, 2012:

Well, I think we're ready: 2-wheel walker, toilet safety frame, bath seat with back, bed bar assist handle—all on three-month loan from the Red Cross. Everything is assembled and in place. We're on the Red Cross's waiting list for a proper size wheelchair. In the meantime, we can borrow one from the hospital, says Dienna, one of Ron's self-styled physio "terrorists".

We've practised the transfers from the wheelchair to the car; the wheelchair parking permit is tucked in the glove compartment; and not a creature is stirring, not even a mouse.

Meanwhile Owen is en route home to Dease Lake. He flies from Victoria to Terrace, where he will do a major grocery shop, and finally, get in his Subaru 4 x 4 for the seven hour drive up the Cassiar highway, through the snow, past moose, wolves, foxes, wild horses, and caribou, arriving home to Jen, Gus the dog, and the 2 cats at about 2 am tonight. We were lucky he was able

21

to string together a few days off and a few days of compassionate leave, because the RCMP detachment in Dease Lake is currently short-staffed.

One of the major factors in recovering from a stroke is getting proper sleep so that the brain can heal and replace the damaged circuits with new pathways. I think once Ron gets into his own bed he might go into hibernation for a while, which will be all to the good. Then, two and a half months of outpatient rehab will commence on Monday, weather permitting. Snow is forecast for Sunday.

I will keep you posted on the success of the move home, but I am expecting that Ron will be able to take charge of his own email very soon.

Love to everyone from us, Pat and Ron

December 8, 2012:

Just a quick note to say that the transition from hospital to home seems to be going well so far. However, the excitement of yesterday found us both a little giddy last night, and quite fatigued today. At the moment Ron is catching some well deserved zzzzzz's. I think we will lie low for the time being.

Undoubtedly Ron's rapid release from the hospital was beneficial to his recovery. I remain convinced of this today. However, one of the reasons that his discharge was possible so quickly was that we lived in a wheelchair accessible house. Therefore, I did not have to hire a carpenter to widen doorways or build ramps with railings so that it was possible to get a wheelchair inside our home. Our polished concrete floors made it easy for Ron to wheel himself all about the main floor. In addition, we had an open shower with three separate heads which made it possible for me to bathe Ron free of worry. I know that most caregivers are not so fortunate.

December 10, 2012:

Ron got his official discharge from the Inpatient Rehab Ward. We snipped off his wrist bands and had a hot apple cinnamon drink to celebrate.

In time, our celebration would prove to be short-lived. Unfortunately, the two and a half months of Outpatient Rehab would turn out to be only a preparation for a much more intense, lengthy, and complicated "care" to follow. Many of the lessons in his daily visits to Rehab proved to be introductory at best. There would come a time in just a few weeks when "care" would become a matter of self-preservation and our own improvisation: a desperate period when we would be left on our own. But, for the time being, we worked hard on

Ron's recovery and my on-the-job training as a care-giver in blissful ignorance.

12 – 12 – 12

Greetings All,

While this is not the 12th update I have sent, nor the first of the twelve days of Christmas, I could not help but note the special date. This is the last time this century that we will get to mark such a beautiful synchronicity and it seems an auspicious day to end my updates on Ron's progress. Each day he gets a little stronger. All the signs are good for his making a full recovery. This is what we are working toward—physicians, nurses, therapists, family, friends—and no one is more determined to get better than Ron himself. I want to thank you for your love and support. It really has made a big difference, so please keep sending us those positive vibes. Love and hope are what the Christmas season means to me. And Ron and I have both in abundance.

Pat e Ronaldo

After the holiday season was over, my life entered a new phase. Although Ron was living at home, I continued to benefit from hospital support. He was enrolled in the Intensive Outpatient Program which was run out of the Rehab ward. There Ron's vital signs and medications were still monitored by nurses. His friendly physiotherapists were still in charge of his physical exercise and his re-learning how to walk, how to climb stairs, how to get up off the floor after a fall. Occupational therapy seemed to me less helpful once Ron had been taught how to dress himself with one hand, and how to manage a spoon, a knife and a fork, implements which initially he couldn't identify. This failure was one of the little signs that indicated things weren't quite as rosy as I thought or had been told.

But the important thing was that I still had the support of the "team." I had people to call upon for help, should I need it. And there were afternoon information sessions when I received advice about diet and safety measures, when I was given volumes of 'informative' pamphlets.

Until the middle of March, I lived in a sort of cocoon. While Ron worked out, I was free to sit by myself and read. The only time I was called on to assist was when he needed help in one of the restrooms, although 'they' were hardly that. Ron struggled with the complexity of zippers, buttons, maintaining his balance, shoes and laces, everything he had previously taken for granted in his daily ablutions. I remember spending a lot of time standing outside the bathroom door, waiting for my cue to enter, while staff paraded by me in the hall, going about their daily tasks. I was the target of many sidewise glances. What did they think I was doing? I wondered, as I loitered by the washroom, leaning against the wall with my hands behind my back.

As the weeks passed, more and more people began to recognize me. Often, we would smile at each other, nod, and say "hello." My embarrassment gradually lessened. But my mantra remained the same:

Expect full recovery. Expect full recovery. Expect full recovery.

In due course, though, this mantra would begin to fade, the hope it forecast would disappear in the daily and lonely drudgery of caregiving without support and relief. Unfortunately, as I would subsequently learn from other stroke survivors and caregivers, Outpatient Rehab programs are much too short, and end far too abruptly. I had no idea of the challenges ahead—like many I would feel like I had dropped off the edge of the world.

CHAPTER THREE

No Time for Tears

Given Ron's progress in Rehab, our wheelchair-friendly house, and my own physical strength and good health, Ron was discharged from hospital relatively quickly given the massive damage the brain attack had wreaked on his body and his soul. Three weeks in hospital, a week of outpatient rehab followed by a two-week Christmas break (through which Ron mostly slept), and two and a half more months of outpatient therapy. The end. A standard program even though the stroke had hit his brain stem and proved far more severe than originally diagnosed. I guess we should have been grateful because, from what we were told, he shouldn't have survived a stroke to this "primitive" part of the brain, the part which is in charge of the body's most vital functions: breathing, heartbeat, digestion, hormones and wakefulness.

Thanks to a requisition from Ron's occupational therapist and Owen's generous donation to the Red Cross's Health Equipment Loan (HELP) Program, Owen and I had modified the house to receive him: we had tucked a bed bar between his mattress and box spring; placed a teal blue urinal on his night table; affixed a metal safety frame to the toilet in the ensuite; set a white plastic bath chair in the open shower area; placed a two-wheel walker and a wheelchair, which I had rented, by the door. In the wheelchair Ron would be able to move easily about the entire main floor.

One observation I have often made silently in the years since Ron's stroke, in the company of the hundreds of health care professionals we have been privileged to meet, is that medicine, as exemplified by its best practitioners, is a *calling*. Some peculiar quirk in their makeup has made these special people choose to spend their adult lives helping others. For this we should all be thankful.

To be wholly honest, medicine, nursing and caregiving had never called to me. Authors, books and the realms of the imagination were, and still are, my passion. Nonetheless, I was totally in favour of bringing Ron home to my care as soon as possible. Although I had little inkling that his speedy release was also administratively expedient, I felt he needed to get back to his own bed, to his study, to my cooking, to familiar surroundings, to much needed peace and quiet—hospitals are not tranquil, quite the opposite, they are industrial on a grand scale.

Having him home was essential to his recovery. His full recovery. Of this I had no doubt.

I was confident I was up to the task. I knew I could push a wheelchair and empty a urinal. But the man whose care I was now in charge of was a far different person from the one I had driven to the hospital on the evening of November 19. As Ron himself admitted:

Norman Doidge, in his brilliant book *The*

Brain That Changes Itself remarks: "In all of medicine, few conditions are as terrifying as a stroke when a part of our brain dies" (162).

Here's the problem: How do you tell other people, especially those closest to you, that the person they're conversing with post-stroke is not the same person they used to know? How do you tell them that it's not just a heartbeat you've missed? And how do you convince family and friends that a little piece of who you were has died, has vamoosed, and that you, yourself, are not sure of what's left of you?

And, furthermore, that even you don't know what to expect of the new you. (Ron Smith, *The Defiant Mind*, 2016, p. 47)

To me, the changes in Ron were painfully obvious. My fully enabled, graceful, and athletic husband had become crippled, in body and in spirit. Post-stroke I began to feel more like Ron's mother than his wife. In many ways he was like a child who needed much love, tenderness and round-the-clock care. Simple skills such as dressing, walking and eating became major challenges. He had to chew his food thoroughly and had to be careful when he swallowed. It was not uncommon for him to choke.

He fatigued easily.

He took long naps.

He needed help in the bathroom and in the shower. He could no longer take a bath. Getting in and out of our tub was too dangerous to attempt. If Ron were to fall, I would be challenged to get him back on his feet and he could be seriously hurt.

Ron's physical problems were self-evident, and his OT (occupational therapist) and PT (physical therapist) were working daily to salvage and improve whatever mobility he had left—along with the attention they were providing several other equally disabled patients. The therapists had their hands full. The intensive Outpatient Program ran five days a week, nonstop, at the hospital.

Ron's emotional problems were also obvious. In *The Defiant Mind*, he notes that as human beings we learn how to defend ourselves against extraneous and unproductive sensations. We filter things out. Otherwise, we would be swamped by all the sensory data which constantly bombards us. After his stroke, Ron's protective filters were wiped out. His vision, his hearing, his memories all seemed sharper. Simply put, his brain and the sensations it responded to seemed more acute, more penetrating. The world in which he found himself had changed. He could hear birds singing blocks away. He could see the individual needles on fir trees. The edges on the timbers in our house lost their hard edges or outlines and seemed to be in constant flux. The laws of theoretical physics literally played out before his very eyes.

His startle reflex sharpened. He jumped in response to sudden movements and noises. He was easily agitated or alarmed. He wanted everything around him to be quiet, dead quiet, and under control. His control. His passion for music, a first love, seemed to be subverted. This heightened reflex often caused us both grief as I prepared meals and washed up in our open plan kitchen with its beautiful travertine countertops. According to Ron, I am a notoriously noisy chef. I attack my work with an exuberance that could be described as Biblical:

Make a joyful noise unto the Lord, all ye lands.
Serve the Lord with gladness! Come into his
  presence with singing! (Psalm 100)

Ron became more emotional. A simple item on the news or an advertisement for the relief of children in Africa could make him weep. Conversely, he got the giggles easily and the two of us could often be found, sitting side by side on the edge of our bed, laughing uproariously at something which struck us as totally absurd.

After his stroke I observed Ron's confidence erode. Living inside a body that would not obey his commands was daunting. His sense of self visibly diminished. For me this process was graphically represented when he started answering his email. Only able to use his left index finger to type, he could no longer capitalize letters. His upper case "I" became a lower case "i".

For me, the hardest times to endure were when Ron's right arm or leg would start to spasm as rapidly as a vibrating tuning fork, a condition known as clonus. He would be in extreme pain for as long as the spasms lasted. These happened frequently and I found witnessing his suffering, knowing that there was nothing I could do to help, distressing. As a caregiver, there is no escape, no relief from these moments.

One of the best things I did for myself, something seemingly small that I continue to this day, was to have our pharmacist put Ron's medication in blister packs, or, if you prefer, bubble packs. These are packages of the weekly medications Ron required sorted into days which are then further subdivided into morning, noon, dinner and evening slots. Overseeing this vital function would have been "a bridge too far for me." It was a responsibility I gratefully left for Russell and his assistant, Jacquie. Pushing Ron's pills out of their pre-sorted bubbles always cheers me up knowing that I have not had to do the counting and the sorting. However, it did take me a couple of years to realize that I could simplify the pill procedure even further by using four egg cups to hold Ron's daily doses, popping all the pills out of their bubbles and into their appropriate cup at one go, instead of four. As I say, this might sound like a simple chore, but when a life hangs in the balance, dependent on about a dozen drugs, one becomes more cautious.

On our west coast, the rainy weather and early nightfall which accompany winter encourage healing hibernation. There is little incentive to go out and little to do in the garden. Even golfers often elect to remain indoors. So, the season was conducive to hunkering down and concentrating on Ron's recovery. Monday to Friday we spent over an hour each day travelling to and from Rehab—a drive which took us past Nanoose Bay, whose tidal rhythms had been a part of our lives since we had first settled by the bay in 1971.

In time, shock and fear and adrenaline subsided and gave way to reality. There had been a death in the family. An able-bodied member was gone and had been replaced by someone who was now disabled and in need of all the care I could give. There had been a death, but I didn't have time to grieve. I was too busy providing care and positive encouragement. Now was no time for tears.

Expect full recovery. Expect full recovery. Expect full recovery.

The mantra of the caregiver continued to play in my mind.

CHAPTER FOUR

The Unknown Zone

When Ron first entered the Intensive Outpatient Rehabilitation Program, we had a meeting with his "team"—Elvira, Rehab's head nurse, his occupational therapists, his physiotherapists and Tina, Rehab's social worker. We all sat in a circle which included Ron, Nicole and me and discussed the work ahead. It was heartening to have so many people united in a common purpose—Ron's recovery.

The ten-week program passed quickly. Ron had managed to get his therapy extended, arguing that much of his time at the beginning had been disrupted by the Christmas and New Year's holidays. Each weekday morning, I packed a lunch for us which we later ate in the hospital cafeteria. While Ron worked out in the gym or on projects in occupational therapy, I sat in a quiet spot at a table by the big windows in one of the therapy rooms and spent much of my time reading.

The book that stands out in my memory is William Faulkner's *Go Down Moses*, a collection of linked short stories, which Faulkner himself called a novel. The connections between the characters are not immediately obvious. I remember copying out by hand the passages I found particularly striking—a practice I employ with many of the books I read—and I believe I even drew up a genealogy to trace the relations between the white and black families descended from their common, slave-owning patriarch. Yet I now discover that I cannot find my notes, that they are not where they should be, or, as Ron would say, they are where I put them. Once again one of my filing systems has, for the moment, let me down. Or perhaps their loss is just one of the many distractions I resorted to as my role of caregiver began to take shape. I was finding ways to cope, some not exactly rational. Perhaps I was playing mind games with myself. Hide and seek. There was so much I didn't know about my own brain let alone about someone whose brain had gone through a massive reconfiguration. Or had gone on a walk about. I was beginning to think about Bruce Chatwin's insights into the aboriginal mind and their relationship to nature in his book *Songlines*. I was beginning to realize that caregiving is a reciprocal arrangement.

Being let down, or loss, was the feeling Ron and I experienced when his Intensive Outpatient therapy ended, and he was discharged from the program. We were cut off and left to our own devices.

No more team.

No more support.

Abandoned.

We looked at each other and wondered *what do we do next?*

Like the Israelites in Exodus, we wandered lost in a wilderness, but without a pillar of cloud by day or a pillar of fire by night to guide us.

* * * * *

On my old computer, the Dell Home Edition, which I purchased in 2004, there was a space on the taskbar that used to pop up briefly when I was about to surf the net. It was tagged *The Unknown Zone*.... I was never able to discover how to access this region, how to open its fleeting portal. I couldn't enter The Unknown Zone, so I never found out where it led.

Yet I was intrigued by the term:

Was it the space we dwell in before we are born?

Was it the place we go to when we sleep yet do not dream?

Was it the dark side known to delinquent Jedi warriors?

Was it the unknown frontier in our brain?

Was it the space we go to when we die?

Or was it simply a fictional location in cyberspace, a creation of techno-nerds?

After Ron's stroke I gained access to an Unknown Zone. It was the limbo I found myself in after his stroke, after the emergency, after the brain attack that changed everything.

By the end of his therapy Ron was a long, long way from full recovery, but we decided not to renew the rental on his wheelchair. We turned in our HELP equipment to the Red Cross. Our loan time was up, and we needed to purchase our own bed bar, toilet frame, urinal, two-wheel walker, and a deluxe four-wheel walker, complete with adjustable handlebars, seat, brakes and removable basket. In part, making these purchases felt like admitting a defeat. As I took out my credit card to pay for all the equipment, I was disheartened. I began to suspect that stroke recovery was not going to be a temporary condition only.

Left to our own devices we began to walk. We walked around our Crescent, measuring Ron's progress by the number of houses we passed, by whether we could make it all the way to the mailboxes and back.

We walked and we talked. We talked to the neighbours we met who were invariably full of encouragement and support.

But still we felt abandoned and continued to wonder *what we should do next?*

In late March, while Ron was watching television and I was preparing dinner, he chanced upon a notice of an upcoming meeting for stroke survivors and caregivers that was going to be held in Nanaimo at Beban Park to advise people like us of the resources in the community that were available to them. Thanks to our attendance at this meeting we learned about the Oceanside Stroke Recovery Society whose weekly Friday meetings were held in the St. Columba Presbyterian Church in French Creek, about a thirty-minute drive from our home. We decided to attend. The sun was shining as Ron and I climbed the three steps which led up to the main entrance to the church. Once inside we passed a library-cum-office on our right, walked through a wide hallway with ample room to hang overcoats before entering a large communal room serviced by a kitchen. Here chairs were arranged in a wide circle for Ron and about thirty other stroke survivors to exercise under the supervision of an exercise therapist—Joan.

With music from the fifties blaring out of a ghetto blaster, Joan began to toss bean bags at her charges who were supposed to catch the bags and toss them back. Some people were able to do this with ease. Some, like Ron, made their best attempt with one arm and hand. Others were unable to catch a single toss and often took the bean bag "right on their chests or chins." It was obvious to me that there was a wide range of physical ability exhibited by the group.

They also did arm and leg exercises from a seated position, alternately flinging each leg and arm out or reaching for the sky. Many, like Ron, couldn't move one leg or get one arm and hand above their shoulders. Some sat in their wheelchairs and drooled while one man tilted his head to one side and slept through the proceedings. Once again, I began to think about the stroke platitude—every stroke is different. And once again I was witnessing someone attempting to apply the same routine to a group of individual cases, treating them as if they were all equally able-bodied. They weren't, far from it. And yet everyone in the group struggled on, determined to succeed. And to my surprise, most of them seemed to take what I saw as a failure with good humour. As I looked from face to face, I realized the great benefit to them was not just the effort to attempt the impossible, but, more importantly, the camaraderie they enjoyed.

As a novice caregiver, I had learned something new. There is a bond between stroke survivors; they understand what each other is going through and share a hope of recovery for anyone suffering from a disability. I would leave this first gathering with an awakened sense of Ron's and my relationship and an understanding of belonging to a new community.

After the exercises were over caregivers pulled out collapsible tables, set them up, and rearranged the chairs around the tables so that everyone could sit to enjoy the lunches they had brought. Volunteers prepared coffee and tea. After lunch, the stroke survivors busied themselves with various therapies and crafts. The theme for these changed weekly, running from painting to music to storytelling to personal hobbies such as sewing and knitting or building something to jigsaw puzzles.

For caregivers there was a meeting room, down another hall past the kitchen. Here we could listen to guest speakers or share our experiences with others. In these sessions I learned that some people had been caring for family stroke survivors for as long as thirty years. Most of the caregivers were women; a few were men. One lady had been looking after her mother for nearly twenty years. She had retired from her own job, her own home, and her own life to care for her widowed mother. Most of the caregivers in the Oceanside group were veterans. They had been at their craft for years. Some of them were angry and frustrated.

I found listening to others instructive, but I soon began to realize that my own wounds were too fresh to be able to share others' pain. Also, I was not ready to open up to strangers. I was not even certain what I wanted or needed to say. So, if I wished, I could leave Ron at Oceanside and go off to do grocery shopping or run errands in Parksville. This free time was precious to me for Ron was still too weak to be left at home on his own.

Some of Oceanside's members were severely disabled. One woman was unable to do anything for herself. Her twisted, frail frame was secured in a wheelchair with a support for her neck and head. Although her eyes were open, she seemed oblivious to her surroundings. Unable to do anything for herself, her husband had employed a full-time caregiver, a young woman, possibly from the Philippines, who, at lunch, broke up her charge's food into small pieces and fed them to her slowly, by hand. This trio—the severely disabled woman, her husband and her full-time paid caregiver—were regulars but I don't remember the husband coming to any of the caregiver meetings I attended. I wondered about this for the longest time. In the end I concluded there was only so much pain a person could endure. Obviously, he cared. I couldn't help but consider my own limits.

By contrast, other survivors seemed completely physically fit and were even able to drive themselves to the meeting. It helped me to be able to grade Ron's condition by comparing him to all the other survivors. I began to appreciate how much worse off I might have been. I learned to be grateful for what I had. I doubt this information was as instructive for Ron; he had seen the range of disabilities while he was in hospital. On the other hand, I was shocked. This was not an illness from which everyone recovered. Far from it. Even those who appeared fully recovered could have an 'invisible' handicap, one that made daily life a struggle. For instance, a serious case of aphasia could be terribly debilitating. For six months we attended the group, until Ron decided to write his book. By this time, I think he was getting restless, wanting to search for other rehab options.

We pursued additional therapies—acupuncture, alternative medicine, private physiotherapy and massage therapy. All of them helped somewhat, but none was a total solution. I am especially grateful to Lisa Watson, Ron's massage therapist. Her treatments were always helpful, but, as important, she was the person who convinced Ron that he should get himself to a swimming pool where he could exercise without the fear of hurting himself should he fall.

Fortunately, we live in a community with a Recreation Centre, now called Fairwinds Wellness Centre, complete with a gymnasium, rooms full of exercise equipment, a games room with a snooker table, a lounge and kitchen. Most importantly, the centre has a swimming pool, sauna and hot tub.

As soon as we joined the centre Ron's rate of recovery speeded up, in large part due to the young Irish personal trainer we soon hired. Though separated in age by a couple of generations the two hit it off immediately. Scott and Ron soon delighted in a raucous banter which formed the basis of their communications. The workouts, though demanding, were always fun for both.

While I can't remember all the exercises Scott imagined for Ron's sessions, his 'stick drawings' provided a guide. Perhaps the most important thing was that they were all intended to address Ron's particular weaknesses. Many were walking and balance exercises. He had Ron walk several times around the perimeter of the gym, without any aids. Speed was not important. Then he would have Ron walk backwards (Scott was always at Ron's side in case he stumbled), followed by Ron walking sideways in both directions. First leading with his right foot, then with his left. And he always had him ride a reclined bike for a minimum of five minutes, as well as kick and dribble a soccer ball for several minutes.

For arm exercises Scott had Ron throw a ball, initially only a few feet, then he would slowly increase the distance. He would have him lift weights on a pulley system. It's important to note that all exercises were done for both sides, the good side as well as the damaged side. Towards the end of each session Scott would put on target gloves and Ron boxing gloves and Ron would try to hit the target. Scott moved his hands around so that Ron was forced to redevelop his hand-eye coordination. He used handgrips with springs which he squeezed to develop hand strength. And so on. Scott was a repository of exercises and always had something new to challenge his student. But always, he kept Ron's specific disabilities in mind.

After eighty sessions with Scott, Ron's physical strength, balance and co-ordination were much improved. He could now walk short distances without the aid of a cane or his walker.

All these extra therapies come with a price tag. Those who can afford them can get them. Those who can't are out of luck. Certainly, their cost cut into our savings. What puzzles me is that the government can't see the false economies behind this policy. It's estimated that stroke costs our country about twenty-seven billion dollars per year. Surely early and continued support of recovery would reduce this expense. Regrettably, recovery post stroke is linked to the depth of your personal finances. The blunt truth is that The Unknown Zone is easier to navigate for those who can afford guides.

CHAPTER FIVE
Self Care

Joining the Rec Centre in the spring of 2014 proved to be beneficial for both Ron and me. While Ron worked out with Scott, I took the opportunity to have a cup of decaf coffee and work on the communal jigsaw puzzle that was set out on a table in the games room. Fortunately, there was also a communal pair of magnifying glasses I could borrow. Having not worked on jigsaw puzzles since I was a teenager, I found the activity surprisingly enjoyable. By now I also knew I needed some relief from 'the job', from the pressure of being constantly on-call.

Working on puzzles has all sorts of positive benefits. The jigsaw puzzle, being visual, exercises both sides of the brain, and increases concentration and creativity. It is a type of meditation, inducing calm, slowing the breath, reducing heart rate, decreasing blood pressure and producing dopamine, a chemical in the brain which is chiefly responsible for learning and memory. Working on jigsaw puzzles is quite literally a *re-creation*.

After Ron's workout he and I would head for the family change room where I took off his shoes and put on his Aqua Socks. Once he was set, I would strip off, douse my hair with cold water, put on my bathing cap, grab my ear plugs and goggles and join Ron in the pool. (Experience has taught me that wetting the hair before putting on a bathing cap stops the hair from absorbing chlorinated water, which, after time, damages the hair, reducing it to a brittle tangle.)

While Ron exercised in the water, I swam laps. As I mentioned, I was once a trained lifeguard and had worked my way through university by giving swimming lessons and lifeguarding during the summer months. When Ron was completing his Master of Arts program in Leeds, Yorkshire, I helped support us by working as a sales assistant in the Gem Super Discount Store, and then, in the spring, as a Bath Attendant at the Roundhay Bath, an outdoor swimming pool in Roundhay Park.

For me, there is something primal about swimming. It frees me from gravity, reminds me of my cousin sea mammals—whales, dolphins, sea lions, porpoises, seals and so forth. When I'm in the water, be it in the ocean, in a lake, in a river, or in a pool, I love to dive, leap, turn somersaults, splash Ron and generally goof around. I love this environment which allows me to act like a kid again.

On an unconscious level, being submerged in water could summon up the experience of being in the womb, when we were all constantly bathed in water for the first nine months of our lives, while our ontogeny recapitulated our phylogeny. Or so I like to think. "Ontogeny recapitulates phylogeny" was a biogenetic law formulated in the 1820s which suggested "that the development of the embryo of an animal, from fertilization to gestation or hatching (ontogeny), goes through stages resembling or representing successive stages in the evolution of the animal's remote ancestors (phylogeny)" (Wikipedia).

Apparently, the theory had shortcomings and by the mid-20th century it was relegated to the realm of "biological mythology." But I feel certain that we were all fish once upon a time. When I am in the water, I know it.

After a swim, followed by ten minutes in the hot tub, followed by a shower in the change room, I feel like a renewed person, cleansed inside and out. I remember thinking as we drove home from the Rec Centre after our first day in the pool: *This is going to be good for Ron, but it is going to be equally good for me.* Ron and I still try to make it to the pool three days a week, and, in the years that we have been members, I always feel better after our time there.

My mother once said to me, "Pat, if you don't take care of yourself first, you won't be able to take care of anyone else." This valuable piece of advice has served me well over the years. She also believed, "If you sleep well, you can cope with anything." I happen to know she was right. Tragically she died when I was only thirty-six, but, for a few precious years before her death, we lived within a couple of kilometres of each other, and, for a short time, we shared experiences as caregivers. While my mother cared for my father, who died at home from lung cancer, I nursed Ron's and my very colicky newborn son. While my mother looked after my dying father, I wrestled with a newborn who wouldn't or couldn't sleep.

My mother and I were usually together at some point in the day during this difficult time. At the very least, we talked on the phone. We concluded that caring for the dying was more difficult than caring for a troublesome newborn. While the demands were similar, looking after the dying was the more depressing duty. Each day my father weakened while the baby, although not sleeping, was thriving. The nickname our family physician, David Stronge, gave him was *99th Percentile Owen*, since Owen was always at the top of the height and weight chart for baby boys.

One of the truisms about strokes is that every stroke is different. One of the truisms about caregiving is that every caregiver's situation is different. In my case, I was always grateful that Ron's mental capabilities were not damaged; that his relation to the language was not impaired; that inside his crippled body, the man I knew and loved was still "in there." This is not true for people caring for spouses or family members who may be physically fit, but mentally deficient; for example, people suffering from dementia, Parkinson's Disease, or in some cases, severe and specific brain damage. Or, to cite another instance, some people suffering with aphasia may still be "in there" but they can't communicate. The words they want to use won't come out properly.

To be perfectly honest, now being fully conversant

with the ravages that strokes can wreak, I am glad I haven't had one. I hope I never do. Although, for a married couple, one stroke is a calamity which changes two lives, I would rather be the caregiver than the stroke survivor.

By the time Ron was discharged from therapy and we were left to discover our own survival strategies, we had accumulated enough helpful literature to fill a sizable cardboard box. Most of it I looked at. Some of it I read. All of it, at the beginning, was overwhelming.

Much of the information we received was directed at caregivers. Online there are hundreds of sites for caregivers and I spent some time surfing these. When I finally sat down to write this book, and was going through my files—email files, notable literary quotations, etc.—I found three items I had printed out from the internet: *The Caregiver Survival Questionnaire*; *A Caregiver's Bill of Rights* by Jo Horne; and *11 Tried and True Caregiver Survival Tips* from the Caring Matters Blog. All three were helpful, but I found answering *The Caregiver Survival Questionnaire* taken from David and Rhonda Travland's *The Tough & Tender Caregiver: A Handbook for the Well Spouse* immediately useful. (I have reproduced it here with Dr. Travland's permission.)

The Caregiver Survival Questionnaire

DIRECTIONS: Read the statements and answer YES or NO. At the end, total your YES answers. Your total could be as small as zero or as large as 22.

___Yes ___No   As a caregiver, do you ever wake up in the morning and wish you hadn't?

___Yes ___No   Are you afraid to admit you are beginning to dislike your ill spouse?

___Yes ___No   Sometimes you get the urge to run away and never come back.

___Yes ___No   Do you sometimes wish you would become sick or hospitalized so you don't have to care for your ill spouse for awhile?

___Yes ___No   Do you often have trouble going to sleep at night?

___Yes ___No   Do you sometimes drink too much alcohol?

___Yes ___No   Do you sometimes yell at your ill spouse?

__Yes __No   Do you feel sometimes that your
ill spouse takes advantage of you?

__Yes __No   Do you notice that your spouse
is indifferent to your discomfort?

__Yes __No   Have your friends disappeared
since you've become a caregiver?

__Yes __No   Are you resentful that your sex-
ual needs aren't met?

__Yes __No   Is your ill spouse resentful when
you do something recreational?

__Yes __No   Have you discovered that you
don't have much to talk about with your ill
spouse?

__Yes __No   Have your children and other
relatives stopped visiting your home?

__Yes __No   Are you eating too much or too
little?

__Yes __No   Do you have a lot more aches
and pains and headaches lately?

__Yes __No   Do you fantasize about having
an affair?

__Yes __No   Do you find yourself depressed or in a bad mood these days?

__Yes __No   Have you begun to neglect your personal hygiene?

__Yes __No   Do you find yourself driving more carelessly than before you became a full-time caregiver?

__Yes __No   Are you a full-time caregiver because of your wedding vows?

__Yes __No   When you feel burned out do you feel guilty?

KEY
0–5: *Relatively low caregiver stress*
6–10: *Moderate level of caregiver stress; need relief soon*
11–15: *Severe stress, immediate action required*
16–22: *Extreme stress, beneficial to see a counsellor, need emergency relief or specialized coaching*

I cannot remember when I took the questionnaire. I believe it was two or three years after Ron had his stroke, well after we had established what Tina, our Rehab team social worker, termed the "new normal." I scored five on the questionnaire and was reassured to learn that, according to the above measure, I had relatively low caregiver stress.

"Who takes care of the caregiver?" is a question that every caregiver inevitably asks. Caregiver burnout is common. One lady I know spent fifteen years being the primary caregiver for her partner who ultimately died of cancer. She put her own life "on hold." Until six months before her partner died, she worked full time to support the two of them. Recognizing the disease was progressing she quit work to be at home, although this decision created immediate financial hardship. She didn't know how to manage her stress and often felt unable to comfort her partner. Angry at her inability to cope well, she was often depressed. She didn't have time to replenish her energy and became run down and exhausted. Her energy level was so low that she felt she was dying, too. There are situations where caregiving is a whirlpool that sucks you down and from which there seems no escape.*

---

* There is help available for caregivers, but how much or how little will depend upon where you live. I have included a short reference at the end of this book which I hope will give caregivers in need of help a few tips on places to start.

CHAPTER SIX

"I Need a Break"

In the summer of 2013 Ron began writing *The Defiant Mind*. His working title was *Rabbit Has Brain*. The A.A. Milne passage which inspired that title is inscribed at the beginning of his book:

"Rabbit's clever," said Pooh thoughtfully.
"Yes," said Piglet, "Rabbit's clever."
"And he has Brain."
"Yes," said Piglet, "Rabbit has Brain."
There was a long silence.
"I suppose," said Pooh, "that's why he never understands anything."

While Ron pecked away at his computer in his study, piecing together his bombarded brain, making something beautiful out of something devastating, I retreated to my study to continue work on a book of my own.

During the space of three decades I had managed to get three books published—*The Golf Widow's Revenge*; *Double Bind*; and *A Song for My Daughter*. My original intention for *Song* was to write a comic novel using the working title, *Double Cross*. It was supposed to be a comic quest novel. Years later, when it was finally finished, I discovered the joke was on me—my heroine revealed herself to be a salmon woman. No surprise there, you may well think, knowing how much I love to swim. Unfortunately, salmon, as far as I know, lack a sense of humour.

Undaunted, I returned to my writing, to tilt once again at my own windmills, trying to write a truly comic novel, tentatively titled *On the Fritz*. This time round I was more confident of success. This time my heroine herself had a sense of humour. How could the *Chimp with a Human Brain* not have?

After writing in the morning and after eating lunch Ron would retire to our bedroom to nap while I would head outside to work in our garden and private forest. Each day Ron would eat, write, eat, nap. Each day I would help him bathe, help him dress, set out his pills, cook breakfast, clean up the kitchen, do the dishes, tidy the bedroom, make the bed, brew tea for Ron, coffee for me, write, prepare lunch, clean up the kitchen, do the dishes, garden.

By the summer of 2013 our lives had settled into a quiet, daily routine.

One of Ron's and my main goals in siting our house was to fit it into the natural contours of our property, while saving as many trees as possible. What I failed to appreciate during the design phase was how much work it would take to keep our driveway, courtyard and terraces looking natural, and not buried under the significant fall of pollen, leaves, branches, needles and fir cones which the trees continued to drop as they lived, grew, fed, communicated and reproduced, all the while replenishing the forest floor with their detritus. The trees did not make any distinction between natural terrains and our driveway, courtyard, patio, water feature, terraces or roof. All were equally blessed. Nor did they appreciate that there were no longer two of us able to garden.

In *The Defiant Mind* Ron refers to the Japanese practice of *Shinrin-Yoku*, or Forest Bathing. The Japanese believe, and science confirms, that spending prolonged periods surrounded by trees is good for human health. Being in the presence of trees reduces the stress hormone cortisol, increases the immune defence system, enhances cerebral blood flow and improves mental health. I know that being outside every day, cleaning up and raking certainly helped me. While Ron slept, I bathed in a forest.

Our lives were quiet, but we continued to believe that Ron would someday achieve full recovery. We were both confident of that. Perhaps that is why the first anniversary of his stroke proved to be such a depressing day. One year out we had expected he would be much further along with his recovery. His right side was proving unexpectedly recalcitrant. The second anniversary of his stroke was less depressing. Perhaps our expectations were lower. By year three, I don't even remember paying any special note to the passing of his stroke anniversary. By this time caregiving had become a part of my daily ritual. Seven years later the anniversary came and went without my even noticing it.

* * * * *

On the New Moon of July 4th, 2016, shortly after the rain let up, I rushed outdoors to finish pruning the young fir tree I had been working on. Earlier, a downpour had forced me indoors. I climbed up my wet, wooden step ladder, reached up with my long clippers and snipped off the remaining unruly sprouts at the top of the tree. Excited to see how the tree now looked, I jumped down off the ladder, ran towards a nearby spot to get the best view, and slipped in a fresh pool of rain water that had collected in a concave dip in a boulder which formed part of one of our many rock terraces. My feet shot straight out from under me and flew up in the air above my head. To cushion my return to the wet rock, I shot out my left hand to brace myself and broke my wrist when I landed.

Until that moment I had never broken a bone and had always assumed that breaking a bone must be the most painful injury a human being could endure. The scream I let out on impact suggested the truth of my suspicions. I picked myself up, cradled my newly deformed left limb close to my breast, dashed around to the main entrance of our house and pushed the doorbell with my right elbow.

Ron answered shortly.

"Call Barb," I instructed. "I've broken my wrist."

I am fortunate to have two sisters-in-law named Barbara. Luckily, the Barbara who lives nearest to us answered her cell phone and was able to cut short her business in Parksville to come and pick me up and take me to Emergency in Nanaimo. En route, resting my arm on the pillow she had thought to bring along for my wrist, I was surprised to discover that I no longer felt any pain. Had I been wrong about the agony I had associated with broken bones? Or was I in shock? According to Barb, I looked as white as a ghost.

Once again I found myself in the waiting area of Emergency at the Nanaimo Regional General Hospital. Once again the wait was about three hours. After an X-ray and subsequently being put under while a doctor and a couple of assistants reset my wrist, I wakened a short time later with a small white plaster cast on my lower left arm. The break had been a clean one. Barb was still with me, waiting to take me home. Six weeks later the cast came off and after a lot of sculling in the pool (making figure eight movements with my hands while swimming on my back) I was once again right as rain.

After nearly four years of being the able-bodied member of our duo, the one who did all the driving, did all the shopping, did all the cooking, paid all the bills, and so forth, the one who had to keep herself fit in case of another emergency, I believe that, without consciously thinking about it, I had begun to sigh and recite under my breath:

I NEED A BREAK. I NEED A BREAK. I NEED A BREAK.

My mantra had changed. And a break is exactly what I got.

The caregiver became the patient. Every caregiver will have these moments when they will depend on the help and support of others. No one is superhuman. Everyone at some point needs love and compassion.

Happily, our kids came straight to the rescue. Owen and Jen were now living nearby on Quadra Island while Nicole, Iain and Flora had moved to Victoria. Both Owen and Nicole were close enough to come by regularly to cook and to clean. Thoughtfully they also came armed with homemade dinners for our freezer. Fortunately, my break wasn't serious. Within a couple of weeks, I was able to drive and manage the basics myself.

There were some notable things I still could not do. I couldn't comb my hair properly, I couldn't put on make up, I couldn't do up a brassiere, I couldn't garden, etc. In short, the regular rituals of my life were suspended, and I got the break I needed. Often, I just sat and did nothing and thought nothing. I got a good dose of respite care, albeit of my own making.

During my "time out" I had a lot of time to think and reflect about my altered situation. I came to appreciate how fragile a human being I really was.

There is an ancient Taoist saying which states that "all things begin in rest." While my wrist healed, I rested and recharged, a thought every caregiver should keep in mind. Perhaps, unknowingly, I was also preparing for the adventures to come.

CHAPTER SEVEN
Family, Friends, Community

Ron and I had moved to Vancouver Island in the summer of 1971 after both of us had spent a year in Graduate Studies at UBC. Ron had completed his first year towards a Ph.D in English Literature while I had finished the first year towards a Master of Arts in Comparative Religion. Ron decided that he needed to take a breather from his studies. Earning some money to repay his student loans was another good reason for a hiatus. He applied to two colleges and one university and received three job offers. We decided to accept the position at Malaspina College where he was hired to establish a Canadian Literature program. Being on Vancouver Island also allowed me to commute regularly to Vancouver while I finished my degree. Our intention was to stay for a year or two, but two summers living in a cabin on the beach on Nanoose Bay changed that. We "came for a day and stayed for a lifetime."

My point is this: Ron's and my connection to the Nanaimo, Lantzville, Parksville and Nanoose Bay area is long-standing. Our roots in the communities are deep. Had this not been the case I know that Ron's recovery would have been even harder and my new role as a full-time caregiver much more onerous. Being able to go out for early dinners on Friday nights with our long-standing friends, Ian and Virginia Garrioch, fed our spirits as much as our stomachs. The fish and chips at the British Bobby were excellent, but Ian and Virginia's company was much more nourishing.

I have long believed that people's senses of themselves, their identities, are, in large measure, something given to them by other people and by the society in which they are raised. Our identities are, in large measure, a gift. (Or possibly, a curse.) Dinners with friends or chance meetings with other people in the community—people who already knew us—greatly helped Ron and I reconnect with our pre-stroke selves and encouraged our healing.

Recent research conducted by the Heart and Stroke Foundation has shown that stroke survivors continue to want and need ongoing support. In this they differ significantly from heart patients who usually feel completely recovered in a couple of months; in most cases, heart patients are ready to resume their lives where they left off without further assistance.

If you are a stroke survivor or their caregiver and have lived in the same community for a long time, much of the support you need is already built in. Nonetheless you will still feel lost. That is why the phone call we received from Linda Ferron in the summer of 2013 was so important. At the time Linda held the unique position of Stroke Nurse Educator at the Nanaimo Regional General Hospital. She had spoken at the information meeting held at Beban Park in the spring of 2013 where she and Ron had initially met. Later, the thank-you letter that Ron wrote to the doctor who had been in Emergency the night of his stroke, whom he credited with saving his life by convincing him to remain in hospital for observation—that letter had been shared with all the hospital staff involved in acute stroke care. Ron's letter suggested to Linda that he would be a good person to invite to assist her in her work. When she called us, she was immersed in developing patient involvement in bettering stroke care at the hospital.

Would we be interested in helping? she asked.

We would, we said, and agreed to meet her at the hospital cafeteria.

Over coffee our feelings of loss, abandonment, and bewilderment gushed out. This meeting was the first time that anyone from the hospital had asked us about our experience. Certainly, it was the first time anyone had listened to us. Being able to tell someone who was sympathetic, understanding and encouraging was a great relief. Linda's listening validated our experience.

Being heard, in and of itself, is therapeutic.

Linda later invited Ron and me, and Michael and Elizabeth Utgaard, to participate in the third provincial Acute Stroke Collaborative that was held in Vancouver in September. Stroke teams from hospitals throughout BC attended. Michael and Elizabeth spoke in front of the entire collaborative about Michael's stroke and their subsequent experience. When the Collaborative divided into its constituent groups, Ron and I met with the Acute Stroke Team from the Nanaimo Hospital. As soon as Ron attempted to speak about his stroke he began to cry. Once his tears came, he could not stop them, and in the end, he was unable to speak at all. In retrospect, I suspect his being overcome by his emotions was more eloquent than anything he might have said.

After the Collaborative concluded Ron and I met Dr. Noreen Kamaal, an engineer who was (and is) "all about improving health care," and Pam Aiken Ramsay, who was the Provincial Director of Stroke Services BC under whose auspices the Collaborative was held. Both women subsequently endorsed and helped promote *The Defiant Mind*, becoming friends in the process.

Pam invited Ron and me to participate in the next Stroke Services Rehabilitation Collaborative: The Journey of a Hero. The format for the collaborative was the brainchild of Cheryl Mitchell, the Collaborative Facilitator. We attended the first learning session on October 29 and 30, 2015 and the fourth and last learning session on November 14 and 15, 2016. Ron's book had been launched that fall and Pam invited him to open both days of the final Collaborative with a reading and a talk. In less than three years, Ron had progressed from being unable to speak about his stroke experience to the ten-member acute stroke team from Nanaimo, to addressing a packed ballroom of health care professionals from all over BC in the downtown Marriott Hotel in Vancouver.

Cheryl took the title for the collaborative, *The Journey of a Hero*, from an article written by Tom A. Hutchinson, then of the Departments of Medicine and of Epidemiology and Biostatistics at the University of McGill, which was published on May 30, 2000 in the *Canadian*

Medical Association Journal. In this article Dr. Hutchinson suggested that approaching patients using the template of the heroic quest was a powerful tool for galvanizing the human spirit. By viewing illness as a story we tell about our experience with disease, the hero's journey provides a structure to transform that journey into a meaningful experience. Although calling patients heroes might not fit with the common conception of a hero as an "extraordinary person who changes the world" it is an apt description for an ordinary person who, as Christopher Reeve says in his autobiography, *Still Me,* "finds the strength to persevere and endure in spite of overwhelming obstacles."

Certainly, as George Lucas demonstrated by the immense popularity of his *Star Wars* movies, there is a little Jedi warrior in us all, asking to be let out. Lucas was influenced by Joseph Campbell's book *The Hero with a Thousand Faces.* In this seminal work Campbell compared myths from around the world and demonstrated that, although the time, place and characters changed, the myths all had a similar structure. The journey of the hero traced and retraced a singular, archetypal structure. Paralleling the stroke victim/survivor's story with that of a hero was instructive and exciting for the entire collaborative. For, like the heroes and heroines who must separate themselves from their Ordinary World and descend into an Other World, pass several tests and trials, find allies, defeat enemies and demons, both inner and outer, before winning the magic elixir that will help them re-enter and change their Ordinary World, stroke survivors must make a similar journey—one that their caregivers share.

Once life goes sideways, things are never the same again. The future you had worked so hard for is never going to be possible. You will have to give up your dream home and most everything associated with it. But, if you open yourself to the experience post-tragedy, if you remain present and compassionate, the undertaking ahead can still be full of adventure. Of possibility.

I kept a record of many of the adventures that happened to Ron and me after the publication of his book in a blog I called *The Defiant Mind Journal*. I have reproduced much of the journal in Part II of this book, which I have entitled "The Hero with a Thousand Faces." Where appropriate I have added new sections to the original blog entries that describe some of my private encounters and thoughts not included in the original text but which I feel are relevant now.

PART TWO
The Hero with a Thousand Faces

Life is full of serendipitous happenings. An idea here sparks a phone call there. A connection is made. A chain of linked events begins. If Ron had not chanced upon the announcement of the upcoming meeting for stroke survivors to be held at Beban Park while he was watching television, shortly after completing his Outpatient Rehab, we would never have known to attend. If we hadn't gone to Beban, we might never have met Linda Ferron or Kathleen Falvai. If we had not met Kathleen, we would not have joined the Oceanside Stroke Recovery Society. If we had not met Linda, we would never have participated in a single stroke collaborative. If we had not attended the first collaborative, we would never have met Pam Ramsay or Noreen Kamal. In sum, most of the adventures that I recount in this section would never have happened. We would never have met all the people who, in their ordinary lives, have become *heroes and heroines*—people who daily find the strength to cope with daunting challenges. Together they total *A Thousand Faces*.

NOTE: In Part Two, the original blog entries are presented in a sans serif font (like this). Afterthoughts are in the serif font used throughout the rest of the book (including most of this note).

NEW BOOK LAUNCHED!

On the afternoon of September 9, 2016, *The Defiant Mind: Living Inside a Stroke*, was launched at the MacMillan Arts Centre in Parksville, BC. The launch was jointly hosted by the publisher, Ronsdale Press of Vancouver, and the Mulberry Bush Bookstore of Parksville and Qualicum Beach.

There were forty people in the audience. Ron was at his ad lib best, reading a passage from his book, talking and answering questions, sitting on a chair at the front of the gallery. There were paintings on the walls, a grand piano in the corner to Ron's left, a cool ocean breeze wafting through the room, sunshine gleaming through the open windows and a congenial feeling emanating from the attentive audience—former colleagues, friends, members of the Oceanside Stroke Recovery Society, and interested readers from the general public.

After Ron's reading, coffee, tea and cookies were served while Ron signed copies of the book.

We had taken our first steps in what was to become a busy fall.

One member of the general audience was a man who arrived in a motorized wheelchair. He sat in a semi-prone position and manoeuvred his vehicle to the back of the room using controls on the arm of his wheelchair. A woman, an attractive and attentive blonde who turned out to be his wife, accompanied him. At the end of Ron's reading, she took command of the question period (I think caregivers often become emboldened when they assume responsibility for someone they know is at a disadvantage and for whom they want to balance an off-kilter world) and then led her husband through the chairs to where Ron was signing books at a table.

"Wheelchair coming through," she announced in a voice which suggested that she was accustomed to taking charge.

People made way, pushing chairs aside to clear more room. After manipulating his wheelchair to the front of the gallery, the man engaged Ron in conversation using a computer-generated voice which sounded only slightly more natural than Stephen Hawking's. The man knew he was difficult to understand so he spoke slowly and deliberately.

While Ron and the man talked, I chatted with his wife. I learned that her husband, who measured six foot five inches tall, had been a veterinarian in the Cariboo. At the time of his stroke he was in his mid-fifties. His catastrophic brain attack had left him totally "locked in." For two years! His body and facial muscles were paralyzed, but he had remained conscious and retained the ability to perform some eye movements. He had spent a lengthy time recovering at the G. F. Strong Rehabilitation Centre in Vancouver. The man and his wife had recently moved to Vancouver Island, settling somewhere near Qualicum Beach.

I admired the two of them. I was awed by the magnitude of their accomplishments.

How had they found the strength of mind to cope? To continue to cope?

Jean Dominique Bauby, the author of *The Diving Bell and the Butterfly*—his heartrending account of being "locked in"—had lived for just over a year after his stroke, dying two days after his book was published. This man had survived for two years and was seemingly going from strength to strength.

How had they prevailed?

I wish now that I had had the foresight to get their names and contact information.

During our brief conversation the woman asked me what types of therapy had been the most beneficial for Ron. I immediately suggested they head for the Ravensong Pool in Qualicum Beach. They had already thought of that, she said, but there was no means of getting her husband safely into the water. He would require at least two able-bodied men to achieve the feat and even then, it would be difficult, if not impossible to do safely.

I hadn't considered those obstacles. Our pool had gently sloping stairs with a handrail which Ron was now able to negotiate on his own. And Ron was able to walk, albeit carefully, with a cane. A pool we would visit later in Creston, a small town in the middle of BC, had a ramp descending into the water for wheelchairs— what insightful designer or community had foreseen this need?

After his reading Ron was surrounded by other people who wanted their books signed, while old friends, many of whom I hadn't spoken to for years, also wanted to talk. In the convivial commotion the man in the wheelchair and his wife slipped away. Their departure unobserved by me.

What I'm certain of is that this man had the will to prevail, no matter what; he wouldn't accept any limitations. But equally important, he had a caregiver whose spirit rivalled his own; she, too, would never give up.

THE TRIP TO EDMONTON

Dr. Noreen Kamal invited Ron to be part of the QuI-CR (Quality Improvement and Clinical Research) DTN (Door to Needle) Collaborative Closing Celebration held in Edmonton on September 23. He was one of two stroke survivors invited to address the collaborative about their stroke experience. As Ron and I learned during the day long session, the Alberta Stroke Program is right to celebrate. They are now world leaders in stroke treatment and care. All Albertans can expect to receive medical attention for an ischemic stroke (a stroke caused by a blood clot in the brain which accounts for 87 percent of all strokes) within sixty minutes if they live in a rural part of the province and within thirty minutes (give or take a few) if they live in a larger centre.

"Door" refers to the door of the hospital and "Needle" refers to the needle which administers tPA (tissue plasminogen activator), commonly called "the clot-busting drug."

These phenomenal times have been achieved by re-engineering the delivery of stroke care. Since "time is brain," the quicker a stroke victim can receive treatment, the more likely they are to suffer minor brain damage. The resulting savings to health care systems are HUGE. And the need for or role of volunteer caregivers suddenly changes.

Instead of using a linear model for the delivery of care, where step A follows B follows C, etc., the stroke teams in Alberta now "swarm" a newly arrived stroke patient, with neurologist, emergency room doctor, CT technicians, admissions staff, all on hand to collaborate, saving precious time. Further brain damage is prevented (and often reversed), thereby dramatically reducing hospital and rehab times. And should a CT scan reveal that a stroke patient needs further intervention, an Albertan can expect to receive the latest revolution in stroke care, an endovascular thrombectomy, whereby a stent is sent through the groin, into an artery, up into the brain, to attach to the clot and pull it out. In some cases, the effects of the stroke are immediately reversed. This procedure is only given if the drug doesn't work. Most significantly, the success rate is close to 70 percent.

People can return home, supported by home care teams, to their families, their familiar surroundings, and their jobs. There are huge savings for the Canadian economy here as well.

Aside from seriously thinking about moving to Alberta, Ron and I were left to marvel at the advancements in stroke treatment being made in the province by legions of inspired health care professionals. And we could only wonder *what if this kind of care had been available for Ron?* And all the other patients we'd met in rehab.

Although BC has a long way to go before it can boast of the stroke care that Alberta provides, important steps are being taken. Endovascular thrombectomy is now performed at four hospitals in BC—Vancouver General, Royal Columbian, Victoria General, and most recently at Kelowna General. Happily, endovascular thrombectomies are even performed worldwide. And Dr. Michael Hill and his global colleagues continue to discover promising new stroke treatments.

BUZZ BOOK T42
Day One

Ron and I have arrived in Washington, "The Ever-
green State." We have crossed through the Peace
Arch, we have our travel insurance documents secure in the glove compartment (who wears gloves
anymore?) and we have just received a shock. Tacoma, the site of the Pacific Northwest Booksellers Association Fall Tradeshow, is *south* of Seattle,
and not *north*, where Everett appears to be. We
will have to pass through the heart of downtown
Seattle! This is an unsettling thought, given that
traversing elevated urban freeway corridors, with
six lanes of traffic going in one direction and six
lanes going in another, is not what I, a resident of
Nanoose Bay, BC am accustomed to. Prior to my
becoming his caregiver, Ron did most of the driving. This is another of the radical changes in our
roles.

But not to worry. There has been a collision on
the freeway near Everett and traffic in all lanes, north
and south, has slowed to a start-stutter-stop pace,
and we have ample leisure to contemplate routes
and roots and exits. Four hours later we work our
way through the American Dream-cum-nightmare
and arrive at Exit 129 in South Tacoma.

I wonder what Chief Seattle would think of his
land now. Was he thinking of traffic jams when he
reputedly said: "Man did not weave the web of life;

he is merely a strand in it? Whatever he does to the web, he does to himself'"?

At the Hampton Inn and Suites, we are instantly greeted with a panoply of peoples. There is a convocation of a dozen or so black ladies of varying ages in colourful dresses celebrating a special occasion, and groups of families conversing in Spanish. At the elevator we are greeted by eight youthful white couples dressed to the nines (whatever that means). The men are handsome in military dress regalia. The insignias and stripes I cannot decipher. The women are gorgeous in long gowns, high heels and elegantly coiffed hair.

We enter the now vacant elevator, press 2, and wait expectantly. Nothing happens. Eventually we see the sign that tells us we need to use our room key to activate the elevator. Once inside our room, Ron stretches out on the bed and channel surfs, amazed to discover the incredible number of college football games we could tune into.

Day Two

The Tradeshow is in the heart of downtown Tacoma in the chic Hotel Murano. Ron and I have arrived at the hotel via the back roads—south Hosmer, south 72nd, south Yakima, 15th Street, and Broadway. We are calm, having avoided Interstate 5, travelling the quiet streets of residential Tacoma, which, if truth be told, look a bit down at the heels.

We find Ron and Veronica Hatch of Ronsdale

Press in the southwest corner of the Pavilion which houses the Tradeshow. They are with the other publishers who are representing British Columbia with a sizable presence—Orca Books, Harbour Publishing, the Heritage Group of Publishers, Greystone Books, Arsenal Pulp Press, Theytus Books and the Royal BC Museum. (Apologies to any publisher I have missed.)

Ron takes his place on a chair in the middle of the aisle beside the sign announcing Buzz Book T42, *The Defiant Mind: Living Inside a Stroke*. Most publishers have selected one of their titles to be their Buzz Book for the show. It is up to booksellers to get their "passports" stamped each time they visit a Buzz Book. The completed passports will be entered into a draw for a $100 prize. For the next six hours Ron engages booksellers and librarians from Juneau and Skagway in Alaska; Enumclaw, Clarkton, Bellingham, Tacoma, Seattle, Port Angeles, Shelton, Yakima, Leavenworth, Friday Harbor, and Bainbridge Island in Washington; Sisters, McMinneville, Portland, and Hood River in Oregon; Coeur d'Alene, Boise and Moscow in Idaho; and a sales representative from Arcata, California, to mention most of the visitors who talk with Ron at Ronsdale Press's booth. There is a lot of interest in his book because, as Ron states in his Preface:

> Every forty seconds someone in North America suffers a stroke.
> Every four minutes someone in North America dies from a stroke.

Stroke is the leading cause of disability in North America.

At the Tradeshow Ron met a young man, who like the veterinarian from the Cariboo, propelled himself with a motorized wheelchair. He was dressed in green and yellow bold plaid pyjamas with matching slippers and nightcap. The young man was the author of a children's book about a character who wore green and yellow bold plaid pyjamas and who was confined to a wheelchair. I didn't get to speak to him, nor did I get the chance to read his book. For the most part I observed him from a distance, darting about the aisles at speeds which left booksellers and publishers gaping open-mouthed in his wake. He proudly told Ron he was self-sufficient. No caregivers. Some stroke survivors or accident victims feel it is important to assert their independence. I'm not sure this young man had had a stroke. More likely, now that I think of it, a motorcycle was his nemesis. He appeared happy and I was pleased for him. Dependency, which I discourage, can be a crutch and destroy hope and the creative spirit.

DOUBLE TAKES

Yesterday (October 20, 2016) Ron and I left home and headed down island to Victoria where Ron was scheduled to tape two interviews for CBC Radio. Our passage through the secure entrance to CBC was made simple by Bob McDonald, the host of *Quirks and Quarks*, who swiped a card over the electronic door lock and ushered us in. "Thanks, Bob McDonald," said Ron, while I did a double take and thought "So that's who he is. I knew he looked familiar."

We were promptly met by Gregor Craigie, the host of *On the Island*, CBC's Vancouver Island morning show. Gregor showed us into a bright conference room where he invited us to make ourselves comfortable so that Ron could recover from the journey before they did the interview.

Point of clarification: Ron needs to regain his land legs and reorient his senses after driving in a car. Fatigue is a condition from which he still suffers, so I monitor him carefully. I like to believe that he does not need to recover from any terrors or white knuckles instilled in him by my driving. In fact, now, after some practice, when Ron and I drive together, we have become a team: Pilot and Co-pilot. (I'll leave it up to you to decide who is which or which is who.)

Before prepping Ron for their upcoming interview Gregor said, "I started reading your book and couldn't put it down. Having a stroke is not something I usually let myself think about, but I found your book fascinating." After outlining the format for the taping Gregor led us into the larger of the two studios on the premises available for broadcasts. Although there was a window looking out into the entrance and the main office, being in the studio felt like lounging in a warm, dark cave. The walls and ceiling were covered in a black, foamy material, obviously designed to dampen any background noise. After showing Ron the proper distance to keep his mouth from the mike, Gregor asked his first question and the show was instantly underway.

The second interview that Ron did was with Sheryl MacKay for *North by Northwest*. This taping took place at 2 p.m. For this "take" Ron was ushered into a much smaller studio, with no window, and more black soundproofing all about. There was a large instrument board with dials, a desk chair in front of the board, and a single microphone dropping down to mouth height from above. Ron sat down in the chair and donned a pair of earphones. I was given a stool on the side of the "cockpit," a pair of earphones and a plug-in jack for my head set so that I might hear the conversation. Ron had done a couple of interviews with Sheryl in the past, so he was comfortable with this arrangement. The two of them talked for almost forty-five minutes, except for a brief interruption by a young man who had to do the live news broadcast at 2:30 p.m. When he left, Ron and Sheryl continued their conversation. An edited version of their talk aired the following weekend.

During our travels I often heard grim tales of arguments sparked when a formerly enabled passenger attempts to offer untimely and unwanted directions to their caregiver who has become the full-time driver—a charged situation which does not sit easily with the new full-time passenger, nor with the new full-time driver. S/he might not take kindly to critiques. Indeed, some drivers have been known abruptly to apply the brakes after an unwelcome instruction, pull over to the side of the road and state, that unless the *backseat driver* can keep their mouth shut, they had better get out and walk.

STROKE AND DISTANCE

"Stroke and Distance" is the headlining caption for Mark Forsythe's review of *The Defiant Mind* which is the cover story in the new issue of *BC BOOKLOOK* (the online edition of *BC BookWorld*).

This headline is a particularly apt description of Ron. For most of his adult life, he was an avid golfer. Indeed, in my youth, I once penned a little story about a mythical golfer named "Don" and the life lessons I learned in *The Golf Widow's Revenge*.

For those of you who do not golf and are not familiar with the game, the term *stroke and distance* refers to Rule 27–1a, which permits a golfer, when faced with an unplayable lie, to pick up his (or her, as the case may be) ball and return it to its previous resting place. If the golfer decides to invoke this rule s/he will suffer a one stroke penalty and the loss of the distance the ball travelled before landing in the unplayable lie.

N.B. This rule does not apply if the golfer's ball is lost or out of bounds. And it certainly cannot be invoked by the stroke survivor who initially is faced with a seemingly unplayable lie. Unfortunately, in real life, unlike golf, there is no possibility of a "do-over." A single stroke is penalty enough. However, given enough time and distance and continuing recovery, Ron is planning his return to the links.

Being able to golf again remains one of Ron's goals, but only when and if he recovers the use of his right arm. In an email to him, Bonnie Sherr Klein, the author of *Out of the Blue: One Woman's Story of Stroke, Love, and Survival*, remarked that there comes a time when the ascending arc of recovery intersects with the descending arc of old age. I don't know if Ron has reached this point yet, but I do know that one of his achievable goals is someday to meet this remarkable woman in person.

Prior to her debilitating stroke in the summer of 1994 Bonnie Klein was a prominent feminist and filmmaker. After enough time and distance passed, she was able to write her story and she has become an effective advocate for the disabled.

Much of what she discussed about her recovery and living in this world as a disabled person has informed how I read and treat Ron. I do my best to regard him as my equal, to treat him as a wholly competent human being, even though he still needs me to help him dress, put on his shoes and tie the laces. Being physically disabled does not mean that a person is mentally disabled. The disabled need to be treated with dignity. Not to do so, is hurtful and counterproductive. Lack of respect destroys self-esteem which in turn can lead to depression and despair. Whenever possible, emphasize the positive.

RIDING THE WILD HORSE, MEMORY
A Review

This morning I was "housecleaning" my Word documents and made the following discovery—the review of Ron's book which was published in the Vancouver *Sun* and five other major Canadian papers in September 2016. Since the review was published before I began this blog, I thought to reproduce it now.

Ron Smith, *The Defiant Mind: Living Inside A Stroke*
(Ronsdale Press, 2016, 313 pages, $22.95)

Two years ago my father-in-law had a stroke. One day he was fine, talkative, alert and chuffed by his recent prowess at the curling rink. The next morning as he ate breakfast, he began to talk gibberish and was rushed to the hospital. Several small strokes ensued. He never recovered his ability to explain what was going on inside during those heart-breaking final days, a terrifying situation for him and for his loved ones. Even his wife, a trained nurse, knew little about the workings of a brain shattered by stroke. If we had read Ron Smith's *the Defiant Mind: Living Inside A Stroke*, I think we might all have responded differently.

The cover painting, Jack Shadbolt's "Bursting Orb," perfectly evokes the central message of this important literary memoir, that a stroke is not just about physical damage, loss of speech, motor skills, even the capacity to swallow; it's equally, or perhaps more importantly, about what is happening in and to the mind that experiences such trauma.

"Was that really me speaking I wondered. It was my voice; it sounded a lot like an old 78 phonograph record spinning at 33⅓ rpm. The words rolled and bounced around the room like tumbleweed blown on a desert wind. They had no traction, no weight, no body. No meaning. And yet they seemed heavy and thick at the same time. Like toffee or treacle."

Smith's sense of humour and gift of metaphor makes this frightening journey into uncharted waters not only instructive, but also very engaging, a work that everyone should read, not only because a quarter of us will suffer a stroke by the age of 80, or be closely associated with someone who has, but also because it's so damn well written.

This book documents loss, confusion, grief and longing, but it's also about a bloody-minded determination to understand the cognitive damage suffered and how that understanding might be crucial to whatever healing and recovery are possible. What seems to Smith the most reliable compass for rediscovering who he is or was turns out to be memory. This is no pleasant stroll down memory lane. Instead, with his body half-paralyzed and senses hyper-alert, Smith rides the wild horse of memory, hanging on for dear life, grabbing hold of unexpected moments from his past, patching together what he can of a lost identity, a Catch-22 process because acknowledging the difference between past and present selves can also be extremely debilitating.

As a writer of poetry, fiction and non-fiction, this must have seemed to Smith very much like the creative process itself, which Joseph Conrad described as rescue work, "snatching the vanishing fragments of memory and giving them the permanence of art." And, indeed, what he has achieved in this epic endeavour—not just dredging the past, but analysing, processing and recording it all on the computer with the index finger of his left hand—is no small miracle; indeed, it's a tribute to the human will and imagination.

Every stroke is different, Smith insists, all the more reason why attention needs to be paid to what is happening to the mind whose "executive function" has been damaged. "Everyone could see the physical damage I'd suffered, and they clearly had some idea of how best to deal with it, but no one appeared to be the least bit interested in my mental state of being. No one asked what my thoughts were or where they led. No one questioned me about the landscape and atmosphere of the stroke world. No one wanted to know its secrets." Happily, with the help of this beautiful, moving and resourceful book, all that could begin to change.

Ron Smith has re-learned how to speak, write, walk, even swallow his favourite treat—apple sauce—but the one thing he refuses to swallow is the idea of giving up.

Gary Geddes, poet, anthologist, playwright, is most recently the author of The Resumption of Play *and* Medicine Unbundled: Dispatches from the Indigenous Frontlines.

What struck me while reading Geddes' review was his awakening sense of his own mortality. Every caregiver is aware of a similar rousing, as if from a deep sleep. Life-altering events bring us up short. Reality shifts cause us to face the ultimate questions of life, death and meaning.

THE JOURNEY OF A HERO
Stroke Services BC
Rehabilitation
Collaborative

On November 14 and 15 at 8:50 in the morning, Ron opened both sessions of Stroke Collaborative #4 with a reading from *The Defiant Mind*. On Monday he read about consoling one of his fellow patients after a rehab session in Nanaimo. At the time, she was feeling extremely depressed because her rehab was not progressing as well as she expected: "Before the stroke I had two heart attacks," she said. "Compared to this they were a piece of cake."

On Tuesday Ron read the opening pages from Chapter 7, "The Wheelchair and the Urinal," which describes his arrival in the Rehab Unit and his initial struggles with the male nurse who was trying to move him from a stretcher to the bed:

> I was terrified. As soon as I was standing, my entire right side collapsed like an accordion. What was happening to me?
>
> "Relax," he said. "You need to trust me. I know what I'm doing."
>
> Trust. This was one of those words I would soon learn was critical to every phase of my recovery. Trust and the need to be brave.

Both Ron and I, and all the other stroke survivors

who participated in the sessions (some in all four) came away heartened to know that the over 100 enthusiastic and dedicated medical practitioners from all parts of the province, from Terrace to the Kootenays, from Prince George to Penticton, from Vancouver Island to the Fraser Valley, are returning to their Health Regions determined to retain the gains in best practices they have made to date, and committed to continuing to improve the rehabilitation of stroke patients. They intend to keep making the best use of the resources they have. In this endeavour they are led by several special people: Pam Ramsay, Cheryl Mitchell and Katie White.

Kudos to all the participants!

I had no idea that what I learned at this collaborative would prove so instructive to me when I came to write this book on caregiving. I could not have predicted that *The Journey of the Hero* would speak to me on so many different levels. Although many people who I met at my table at the back of the ball room suggested I should write a book about my side of the story, my typical response was my wan smile and shrug.

There is no school for caregivers; you learn on the playground like all the other novices encountering disability for the first time. What makes the learning so difficult is that all the lessons are different.

A QUOTE FROM DAN NEIL

January 13th

Ron, I have finished your book and was sad to leave it. I would say it is a beautiful book because anything is beautiful if it comes from our honest creation. An inward-looking book, personal, but so relevant to everyone. Many times I had to stop and consider consciousness, awareness, soul, spirit and stillness. I whole heartedly agree that somehow technology has become our master, that we have forgotten the awesome beauty and potential of the human mind. You're a wonderful writer, Ron, and what a great book.

Dan

Dan is a writer and photographer who lives in the Okanagan. I have quoted Dan because he echoes my feeling of caring for the whole person—body, soul, spirit—inseparably. Caregiving is too often about the body only.

APPLES & BEETS

On Monday, January 16th at 11:30 a.m. Ron and I were navigating the intricacies of "Spaghetti Junction" en route to Ron's first engagement of 2017 with the Saanich Peninsula Stroke Recovery Association. Their meetings are held every Monday from 11 a.m. until 2 p.m. in the Seventh Day Adventist Church which is located on the left side of Willingdon Road just before the roundabout leading to the Victoria Airport. The unique thing about roundabouts is that, if you miss your turn, you can keep going *round about* until you eventually return to the correct exit. This feature was particularly helpful to me as the driver on Monday morning.

Once inside the airy church we were met by the Association's president, Lyall Copeland, and some of the Association's many volunteers. This event was special since it was the first time that Ron was speaking to an audience comprised solely of stroke survivors and their caregivers. One of the principal impetuses behind *The Defiant Mind* was "to write a book that provides a voice for victims," to show that *recovery is possible*, and to advocate for engaging the hearts, minds and brains of stroke survivors, and then utilizing their insights in their rehabilitation programs. After Ron's reading and talk, one gentleman on his way out the door to catch his ride home with a Handy Dart announced to the whole group, "I endorse everything you've said here today, Ron. You've nailed it."

Ron's next rendezvous was at 2 p.m. at the Tim Hortons in the Eagle Creek Centre across from the Victoria General Hospital. Dana Haydon, a speech therapist at VGH, had asked if Ron might be able to meet with one of her patients, Christina Willing. Christina had read Ron's book and was very anxious to speak with him. Christina is a sprightly ninety-year-old, who had her stroke last February, a stroke which left her unable to speak, and who, thanks to her therapists and her six children, (daughter Belle Belsky was the designated driver of the day) has been able to return to her farmhouse home and re-sume her independent life there.

Ron and I returned to our home in Nanoose Bay enriched by our encounters with new people, by a pint of home-canned beets we received from one of the volunteers in Saanich and by a bag of apples from one of Christina's heritage apple trees, the latter gift inspired by the section on apples in *The Defiant Mind*:

> I imagined eating an apple, not whole, but as a warm sauce over ice cream or peeled and cut up and baked in a fine, fluffy pastry crust, served with a slice of cheddar. A yellow trans-parent apple picked just as it turned colour, from a deep lime green to the pale shade of the moon. Not what they used to call an eat-ing apple but a cooking apple. Slightly tart, with a sting in its tail. Not an apple you would feed to a horse but an apple whose juices lin-

gered like the summer sun on your tongue during a fall rain or winter snow storm. An apple that held the reach of a climb when you had scuffed a bare knee against rough bark. An apple with a short ripening season, testing your will to live another year. (p. 123)

Christina Willing phoned just the other day. She calls us occasionally to keep in touch. She is now ninety-three and still lives alone on her fifteen-acre farm outside Victoria. She delights in the flocks of birds that settle on her property, whose antics she observes from her dining room window. When she does go outside, she uses a walker and is careful where she puts her feet. She knows how important it is not to fall if she is to continue to enjoy her independence. In her determination to do this, she is actively aided by her children.

Ideally caregiving should never be the responsibility of one individual; it can include the extended family or an entire community. This depends on the patient. Ron is a private person, so I tend to be somewhat protective of him. Seeking a balance is difficult because I'm gregarious. I've had to adapt since so much of my time now is shared with Ron. Sometimes I'm desirous of what I've had to give up. I don't think I'm being unreasonable. Maintaining connections with friends is essential to a caregiver's well being. But one of the things I still miss is time alone in our home, time when I will not be interrupted.

LITERATURE LIVE

On Sunday, January 22, Ron and I traversed the 49th parallel at the Peace Arch crossing just south of White Rock. We were headed down I-5, bound for Village Books and Bellingham Bay on the Salish Sea. After taking Exit 250 for Chuckanut Drive and the Old Fairhaven Historic District we soon found ourselves amid wide streets with angled parking in front of multi-storey red brick buildings. We located 11th Street and parked in the handicap spot directly in front of Village Books.

It was three o'clock. One hour before Ron's reading. After making the appropriate introductions and sussing out the reading space in the basement, we rode the in-store elevator to the top floor where the cafeteria was located. I noticed that the *Fiction Section* of the store was also located there. Was this by accident or design? I wondered.

While Ron went to get us a window seat, I stood in line for two hot chocolates and two Swedish cinnamon buns. As the hot chocolates were being topped with whipped cream by the waitress, I noticed that I might have ordered a beer from a cooler containing a wide sampling of local craft beers. Beer in a bookstore! What a *novel* idea! I thought.

In a corner of the cafeteria, overlooking Bellingham Bay and the San Juan Islands, two young male guitarists were quietly performing a selection of folk tunes. The room was primarily full of young people, probably students from the University of Western Washington. When Ron and I finished our buns and chocolate we returned to the bottom floor and made ourselves at home.

Members of the audience drifted in.

Conversations began.

At four, a young man named David, who looked remarkably like Harry Potter, introduced Ron. Ron then read from his book and answered questions from the audience which had grown to about thirty people. At half past five, people began slipping away but the conversations continued. Three people had had strokes recently. Some had family members who were still suffering. Others were caregivers or therapists. One lady and her fourteen-year-old son had recently sailed down from Alaska and were living on their sailboat in the Bellingham Marina. Everyone we met was welcoming, helpful and friendly. Characteristics Americans used to be famous for.

Outside, across the street, atop another heritage building, a huge American flag wavered in the onshore breeze. However, as Ron and I now knew only too well, strokes pay no mind to walls, borders, and lines drawn on maps.

On reflection stroke conversations have an eerie similarity to them no matter where in the world you travel. As do caregiver conversations! Recently, on a Baltic cruise to celebrate our 50th wedding anniversary, Ron and I met a Dutch couple, Mel and Toos Beverwijk; he had had a stroke, she was his principal caregiver. Mobility, diet, bathing, fatigue, medications, all the same old subjects came up in conversation. However, Mel had a wonderful scooter that allowed the two of them to take advantage of onshore excursions that they organized themselves. The scooter was lightweight and folded up for easy transport in a car. Meanwhile Ron and I were often stuck onboard. The wheelchair that we had rented was not built to navigate cobblestones and Holland America did not offer any excursions that catered to their many disabled passengers.

WORDS from the WEBSITE

Dear Ron,

One month into my brother's survival of a catastrophic stroke that wiped out his right brain at
age 44, I just finished reading your book today. In a
labyrinth of misinformation, and at times despair,
your words have been the reassuring thread I've
followed. When nurses are mean and procedures
are dehumanizing and terrifying, your words and
your humanity are there providing untold comfort.
Your insights about giving yourself over to the various procedures were particularly helpful—until I
read that I cringed for every imagined "attack" I
knew my brother had to bear. Likewise, your un-
fortunate room-mate—the kind of character a
fictional editor would demand as a hurdle for the
hero, no? But how illuminating to think that the
cranky juice fiend played his own role in you finding your way back.

I want to give every single health professional I
meet this book. I've also read *Stroke of Insight* and
have a stack on Neuroplasticity to follow up on next,
but *The Defiant Mind* is head (both lobes) and shoulders above.

As a writer, I'm in awe of what you've accomplished with this book. How can something so useful
be lyrical!? It's also an incredible inspiration—anyone
suffering a mild case of writer's block should pick up

a chapter and think *I* didn't have to surmount that to set words to page!

Again, thanks. And best wishes that tiny improvements ever continue. Bravo.

—Emily Weedon, January 25, 2017 @ 11:45 p.m.

Emily's story was sad but typical. I remember feeling the same anger and having the same sense of futility. There's nothing you can do. Brain damage is simply not understood, at least not very well. Grief runs from head to toe, so to speak, from the neurologist to patient to family. One of Ron's doctors kept answering our questions with: "I don't know, I've never had a stroke." He wasn't being facetious, just honest.

I continued to take comfort from the responses Ron received from readers of *The Defiant Mind*. Each person had something as unique as their stroke to say. The following words from Doug Watkins humbled me. Stroke survivors choose their words carefully, perhaps because so many of them have had a close encounter with silence.

MORE WORDS from the WEBSITE

IF Tolstoy had written 'Stroke and No-stroke', IF Kilmer had seen no trees, and IF you hadn't written this book, I would be the loser!

Change each word 'Pat' to 'Joy' (my wife's name) (she is my caregiver, too, and has been my wife for more than 50 years). I am 80 and have had a stroke and do go to the 'Y' for swimming and physic, and do belong (& attend) the local "Stroke Survivors" group. I read a lot and just finished your book and I want to thank you.

—Doug Watkins

BACK TO THE FUTURE

DENSE FOG VISIBILITY LIMITED was the warning on the highway sign at the base of the Malahat as Ron and I drove south to Victoria on February 15th. In fact, the warning told us nothing new since we had encountered such conditions for the previous seventy kilometres. From Nanaimo south the fields were still snowbound. A thick mist, caused by warm temperatures and heavy rain, rose from the fields creating the fog.

Ron had been invited by speech therapist Dana Haydon to speak to one of her therapy groups which meets in the Community Room in the Uptown Mall in Victoria every Wednesday. The people who attend this group suffer from aphasia caused by a stroke or other brain injury. Aphasia is the inability to comprehend and formulate language. Intelligence is unaffected, but the people who Dana works with have difficulty reading, writing and speaking. Often, they cannot find the right words to express what they want to say.

As children, it takes us years upon years to learn to speak, to read and to write. Many of the people in Dana's group must go back to basics and re-learn these precious accomplishments. The logic behind the Uptown Mall location is that the group is able to take what they learn in the Community Room and immediately go out into the real world and, with the help of Dana or her fellow speech pathologist,

Janine, put these re-learned skills into immediate use. The powerful message which Ron brings to groups like Dana's is to never give up, to reassure them that healing continues to happen, that it never stops. The gift he receives in return is the warmth, support and gratitude from courageous people overcoming daunting and frustrating obstacles, all of whom yesterday insisted on buying his book, determined they will soon even be able to read it.

One of the most important stroke books I have read is Diane Ackerman's *One Hundred Names for Love*. When her husband, the writer Paul West, was in his late seventies, he suffered a massive stroke which totally bombarded his brain. He was left with global aphasia. Ironically, especially for a wordsmith, the language areas of his brain lost most of their ability to process language. Her husband was no longer able to speak sensibly.

Luckily for Paul, Diane was an accomplished writer herself, and she wasn't prepared to give up on his reading, writing, and speaking. Or their intimate word play. After getting him home from the hospital she hired several different people to help with his daily care and encouraged the help of traditional speech therapists, whose therapies often left Paul frustrated and demoralized.

One day, long after he had been discharged from hospital, she happened to be walking through their home library where Paul was working with a speech therapist. She observed the woman pointing to the telephone and heard her ask Paul to tell her what it was. When Paul responded tentatively with the word TESS-er-act, the therapist corrected him, announcing that he had used another of his nonsense words.

Diane immediately turned around and corrected the therapist. She advised her that *tesseract* was a *real* word. "It's a three-dimensional object unfolded into a fourth dimension. In a strange way, he's right, that's what a telephone is."

Diane "didn't actually mean the fourth dimension of time we associate with space-time, but a physical fourth dimension—like length, breadth, and width . . ."

Paul nodded vehemently in response.

This was the transformative moment when Diane's understanding, Paul's therapy and the trajectory of their lives dramatically changed. Diane realized, as my husband Ron maintains, that a stroke survivor's therapy should focus on his or her strengths and not on their weaknesses. On page 193 of *One Hundred Names for Love* Diane states: "From then on, I began rethinking Paul's therapy and creating homework tailored to his lifelong strengths, words and creativity, exercises with a little fun, a little flair, and not condescending.... Had he been a welder or a golfer, I would have tried to include those activities."

Recovery post-stroke should attempt to tap into the neural networks and connections that have been built up over a lifetime. With engaging and inventive therapies tailored to a stroke survivor's strengths, neural rewiring can be speeded up and healing encouraged. A bridge between the pre-stroke person and the post-stroke person can be built.

In the nine years since Ron had his stroke he is still dumbfounded to know while lip service is paid to the fact that every stroke is different, the treatment and therapies for stroke survivors are still generally the same. The emphasis is always on the stroke survivor's disabilities. These are obvious. Yet the stroke survivor's abilities are never identified and hence never tapped. They are never engaged to aid and enliven recovery. If they were, recovery therapy could extend in all sorts of intriguing directions.

The whole person could be engaged.

Bridges could be built to link the pre-stroke self to the post-stroke self.

Recovery might even, at times, become fun.

And who better than caregivers to help identify the stroke survivors' previous abilities, interests and passions?

Once Diane Ackerman actively took part in designing her husband's speech therapies, his recovery rapidly improved.

He went on to write several more books.

The lesson here is clear:

We need to stop treating the part.

We need to engage the whole.

IS AN OCEAN BIGGER THAN A LAKE?

Each time that Ron is asked to speak at a Stroke Recovery Group we are reminded of the tremendous physical and mental devastation that strokes can cause. As Dr. Michael Hill states in his introduction to Volume II of *Brain Attack: The Journey Back,* "Recovering from a stroke may be the hardest thing one can ever do in one's life...."

A copy of Volume II was given to Ron last Friday, March 31, by Dr. Alvin Yanchuk at the weekly meeting of the Victoria Stroke Association in the Knox Presbyterian Church. Dr. Yanchuk is a stroke survivor and a senior scientist in forest genetics with the British Columbia Forest Service. On March 20, 2015, at age 57, he had a stroke which left him unable to swallow, speak, read or answer the question, "Is an ocean bigger than a lake?"

Two years later he can do all the above and his recovery story is one of many featured in Volume II. Although Dr. Yanchuk's physical body was left mostly unimpaired, except for issues with his balance, he had to learn how to speak all over again. Simply being able to pronounce letters such as 'k', 'g' and 'z' took him months.

Prior to his stroke Dr. Yanchuk "wrongly assumed" that strokes "only happened to people who did not take proper care of themselves." He had been in good shape all his life, playing hockey and basketball, practicing karate, running, hiking and fishing. Now he realizes that EVERYONE "is a potential stroke victim." Even today his doctors cannot say exactly what caused his stroke. However, he has learned that with luck, hard work and professional help, he can get close to being his normal self. That remains his goal. And, from what Ron and I observed last Friday, as he was leaving the meeting early to go to work, he was well on his way to doing just that.

"WOMEN HELPING WOMEN"

Since 1987 the Peninsula Newcomers Club has been welcoming women who have recently moved to the Saanich Peninsula. Their motto is "women helping women." (It seems the married men are left to fend for themselves, although they do get to share in the occasional dinner out, for example.) The club organizes activities to appeal to the chefs, the thinkers, the readers, the hikers, the adventurers and the artists in their midst.

Nonetheless, the emphasis of the club remains on the NEW. After five years (or optionally after four) a club member is expected to be fully integrated in the community and must graduate in June. In this manner the club ensures that the membership and the executive are continually changing and re-charging.

Every second Thursday, from September to June, the full club contingent of seventy ladies lunches at Haro's Restaurant in the Sidney Pier Hotel. The Sidney Pier itself is completely visible from the picture windows in the seaside dining room. While the ladies are enjoying their dessert, they are treated to an after-luncheon speaker who talks on a subject deemed to be of interest to the members, which is why Ron was invited to last Thursday's lunch. (Ron's sister-in-law, Barbara Osaka is a home care nurse, and her sister, Pat Montgomery is a member of the club. Having both read *The Defiant Mind*, the sisters agreed that inviting Ron to address the Newcomers Club would be a good idea.)

The event was unique for Ron in a couple of ways: It was the first time he had ever been an "after-dinner" speaker. In the early months and years after his stroke Ron found eating out disorienting. The clattering of plates and cutlery, the noise of different and simultaneous conversations, the hustle and bustle of waiters, all of the general hubbub in a restaurant which most of us take for granted and unconsciously tune out, can be overwhelming for a stroke survivor who has yet to re-learn this skill.

It was also the first time Ron had ever addressed an all-female gathering. Perhaps this is why he began his talk by recalling the moment when his stroke finally hit with massive force in the waiting room in the Emergency Department of the Nanaimo Regional General Hospital on November 19, 2012. After sliding off his chair onto the floor as his orb exploded, he was whisked into a treatment room where "the next thing I knew my clothes were being removed. Shoes and socks first. I didn't have to lift a thing. My rear end and legs were raised, my pants came off. My torso sat up, my arms rose above my head and my shirt slipped off. . . . 'Aren't you a lucky man,' the head nurse said, 'you've got five women undressing you.'"

"Every event has its right moment," he said. "This wasn't one of them."

One of the enduring side effects of Ron's stroke remains his sensitivity to noise. I continue to be a noisy cook and Ron's sensitive startle reflex continues to plague him. Eating out at a restaurant is no longer a prospect that appeals to him. It still appeals to me, though, and I continue to dine out at lunch with friends whenever the opportunity arises. What I'll give up for caregiving has limits.

IPPY GOLD MEDAL for THE DEFIANT MIND

Some days are full of happy surprises. Today was one of those.

CELEBRATING INDEPENDENCE

Especially around the 4th of July, it's fun to draw comparisons between independent publishing and the American Revolution. Colonists vs. the British; Patriots vs. Loyalists; Indie publishers vs. Big Five trade publishers; Indie bookstores vs. Amazon—the skirmishes continue. Yes, independent publishing is a revolutionary act, and it's a battle under the best of circumstances. But sometimes tragedies occur that make it even harder.

This month's feature article, Once Upon a Time an Author Had a Stroke, began as a review of the IPPY Award-winning memoir, *The Defiant Mind: Living Inside a Stroke*, the story of long-time Canadian author Ron Smith's slow recovery from a massive stroke in 2012. While corresponding with our reviewer Anita Lock about the book, his answers were so compelling that we decided to include their conversation and turn it into a feature story. "(The book) took me over a year and a half to write, pecking one letter at a time with the index finger on my left hand..." begins Smith's tale of his ordeal. It's heartbreaking to picture his recovery efforts,

but uplifting to recognize his strength and spirit—
especially when you realize the motivation is to assist
other stroke victims and their caregivers, and even
to shed light on the workings of the brain for health
professionals with his insightful observations. It is an
honor to have awarded this book a gold IPPY medal.
And very humbling to observe his determination
and perseverance.

—Jim Barnes, Editor and Awards Director,
Independent Publishers, USA

The day the gold medal arrived from Ronsdale Press
Ron told me we shared this award. Most of the time
we are a good team but sometimes he feels that he is a
burden. And often my caregiving duties feel onerous.
The continuing trick for both of us is to remain positive.
And for me to remember that caregiving, ideally, is a
gift given, unconditionally.

THE WHEELCHAIR and THE URINAL

On Thursday, April 27th Ron was invited to speak to hospital therapists, nurses and administrators who work with stroke patients in Victoria. Two sessions were scheduled for the day—the first one in the morning at Royal Jubilee Hospital, and the second one, in the afternoon, at Victoria General Hospital. Both sessions were well attended with approximately sixty people crammed into the lecture room at Royal Jubilee, and approximately fifty people at VGH. A few people attended both sessions and the feedback Ron received was excellent.

His presentation to both audiences was substantively the same. He opened his talks with a reading from Chapter Seven of *The Defiant Mind* entitled "The Wheelchair and the Urinal." This chapter recounts Ron's arrival on the Rehab Ward of NRGH (Nanaimo Regional General Hospital) from the Acute Care Ward on the fourth floor:

> "Don't fight me," he said.
> "I'm not," I said.
> Once again I heard that strangely garbled voice.
> "You are."
> He held me in a modified bear hug, trying to transfer me from the stretcher to my new bed in the rehabilitation unit. Somehow he managed to get me sitting upright on the edge

of the stretcher, then by gaining purchase under my arms he got me standing on two very wobbly legs, at which point I grabbed him with my left arm and clung to him like a bear cub to its mother.

I was terrified. As soon as I was standing, my entire right side collapsed like an accordion. What was happening to me?

"Relax," he said. "You need to trust me. I know what I'm doing."

Trust. This was one of those words I would soon learn was critical to every phase of my recovery. Trust, and the need to be brave.

For people like Ron, who a mere week and a bit before landing on the Rehab Ward, had been a healthy, fully functioning, independent person, able to dress himself and drive his car, a stroke is a bolt out of the blue, traumatizing and brain bursting. The struggle to re-orient one's self in the world with a damaged brain, loss of mobility, and a lost sense of belonging becomes a major struggle. Wheelchairs and portable urinals, although helpful aids, can seem alien and even threatening.

Because of the brain damage that stroke survivors have suffered their perceptions of the world may be radically altered. While some functions are lost, other senses may be heightened, and some experiences can even be terrifying and cause people to feel they are going crazy.

One of the people Ron contacted, after his formal rehabilitation had run its course, was a Dr. Hobson, a neurologist at Harvard University in Boston. Dr. Hobson suffered a stroke while on vacation in the south of France about twelve years ago. Upon his return to the US, Dr. Hobson tried to persuade his Harvard colleagues that the experiences he had had during and post stroke had convinced him that, if the personal stories of stroke patients were recorded and written down, over time there would be enough anecdotal information collected that could provide valuable insights into the workings of the brain. Dr. Hobson's post-stroke experiences, when viewed from the perspective of current scientific knowledge, would have been discounted as the impossible rantings of a lunatic. But, as Ron emphasized in his talk, stroke survivors have extraordinary experiences. He cited the example of the man who, after his first stroke, while watching the Beijing Olympics, had felt himself transported over the television signals to Beijing where he was able to observe the events "first-hand." Of course, his detailed responses to the smells, sounds, atmosphere, movement, excitement were simply dismissed as imaginary. After his second stroke this same man acquired the ability to "taste colours." An ability which researchers subsequently put to the test. They wired up the man's brain and when they showed him different colours the taste centres in his brain continually "lit up."

Every person's story is important but stroke survivors' stories, if taken seriously and recorded, could have much to teach us about the marvel that is the three-pound mystery in the heads of each one of us—the marvel that is the human brain.

We might learn that there is a commonality to the stories, we might learn that there are patterns the stories share, but, most important, we'll know that these people are not hallucinating or crazy.

KUDOS FROM CALGARY

Ron—

It usually takes me weeks to read a book (too busy to read—or too tired!) but I finished yours in a few days. It was so compelling. I have no experience with strokes, so I didn't know much about them. In our family, heart attacks have taken their toll, but not strokes.

I had no idea they were so common or that they caused so many deaths and disabilities. Your personal accounts of the stroke and its repercussions for you and for Pat made me feel some of the pain and agony, frustration and desperation that you went through. It was amazing to read of your recollections when the stroke happened, what you felt and thought. And all the long months of recovery, your persistence, and your passionate will to overcome its effects.

I am very glad that your book has received so much praise and will help the public and the medical profession to understand this disease and the difficulties involved in treatment and rehabilitation.

After reading, I immediately phoned a friend from my outdoor club whose husband has recently experienced a stroke. You will be pleased to know that one of the nursing staff had already told her about it and she had a copy.

Blessings,
Cheryl

Cheryl is my cousin who lives in Calgary. Her husband, Bruce, a lovely man, had recently died of a heart attack while out hiking in the Rockies. I was amazed how closely Cheryl's response to stroke paralleled mine, both of us equally ignorant on the subject. I wonder how many people are as innocent.

THE NEAR and THE FAR

On Friday, May 19th Ron was invited to speak at the Probus Club of Nanoose Bay, a mere five minutes away from our home. The club meets in St. Mary's Church Hall on Powder Point Road at 9:15 a.m. on the third Friday of each month. This social club caters to the interests of a diverse and active membership. Guests are welcome to attend. However, if you wish to join, you will have to put your name on a waiting list until a space becomes available.

After the morning meeting was finished and coffee break over, Ron spoke to the ninety-five members present, his subject in diametric opposition to the jovial, boisterous atmosphere in the Hall. He began by reading a short passage near the beginning of *The Defiant Mind:*

Imagine. Imagine you suddenly see the world disappearing down a tunnel. Darkness surrounds a diminishing circle of light as it recedes into the distance. Light is leaving you. . . . All energy has left you. Your limbs feel limp, your body sags into itself like a bean bag. You begin to slide off the front edge of your chair. Suddenly. Involuntarily. You are in slow-motion free fall. Perhaps it's resignation. Whatever happens will happen. There seems to be an inevitability about this event that you don't comprehend but that you curiously accept. Your body and spirit have been deflated in an inexplicable way. You are experiencing a mystery. And you are terrified.

Ron spoke for nearly an hour to a rapt audience and, when he finished, the applause he received was generous and genuine. One member even gave him a standing ovation.

He emphasized how little we know about the brain, at one point quoting from Michio Kaku's *The Future of the Mind:*

> You may have to travel twenty-four trillion miles, to the first star outside our solar system, to find an object as complex as what is sitting on your shoulders. The mind and the universe pose the greatest scientific challenges of all, but they share a curious relationship. On the one hand they are polar opposites. One is concerned with the vastness of outer space, where we encounter strange denizens like black holes, exploding stars, and colliding galaxies. The other is concerned with inner space. Where we find our most intimate and private hopes and desires. This mind is no farther than our next thought, yet we are often clueless when asked to articulate and explain it.

STROKE MONTH SAGA

It all started innocently enough. Donna Hastings, CEO of the Heart and Stroke Foundation of Alberta, the Northwest Territories and Nunavut, invited Ron to speak at a meeting of her Regional Managers to be held in Calgary on June 8. Ron accepted and Donna suggested he also contact Vicky Jones, President of the Stroke Recovery Association of Calgary. Ron did and Vicky promptly invited him to speak at their annual "convention" on June 10th at 10 a.m. SHARP. Ron accepted. When Betty Jane Hegerat and Tyler Perry heard that Ron was coming to Calgary they arranged for Ron to read at Shelf Life Books on Wednesday evening, June 7th at 7 p.m. or thereabouts.

In the meantime, Marg Dietrich, a facilitator for the Heart and Stroke Foundation's *Living with Stroke* program, had already written to Ron, telling him how much she had enjoyed *The Defiant Mind*, and, with the assistance of Head Librarian, Anne DeGrace, the two ladies arranged for Ron to read at the Nelson Public Library on June 1st at 7 p.m.

I was pleased. This would be a good chance to meet up with my cousin Cheryl. Also, I have always wanted to visit Nelson, for many reasons: My long-time friend, Suzanne, lives in Nelson and I thought that this would be a good chance to see her. Also, I am old enough to be a fan of the movie, *Roxanne*, starring Steve Martin, set in Nelson, and I thought that the reading would give me time to see the city firsthand.

When Deborah Rusch, Manager, Promote Recovery of the Heart and Stroke Foundation in BC, heard that Ron was heading east she suggested that the two of them join forces. Deb would set up "Lunch and Learn" sessions at several hospitals in the BC Interior. Heart and Stroke would provide the lunch. Deb would talk about the Heart and Stroke Foundation's new Living with Stroke program for stroke survivors, caregivers, and other interested parties, and Ron would follow with his personal story and a reading from his book if he were so inclined. He was.

So, on Saturday, May 27th Ron and I packed up our baggage and bed bar and drove to Vancouver to pick up books from Ronsdale Press. After an overnight stay with our good friends, Bill and Peggy, we departed for Kelowna the next morning and our Stroke Month Saga was underway.

My role of caregiver had expanded to that of a 'roadie'.

RETURN to the OKANAGAN

For Ron and me our Stroke Month Saga was the first major road expedition that we had attempted since his stroke in November 2012. It had been eight years since we had headed up the Coquihalla Highway. The first feature that struck me as we neared the Nicola Valley was how green and plentiful the trees were. The last time we had passed this way evidence of the pine beetle infestation was everywhere. The orange and dying boughs on most of the pine trees suggested that this forest was in trouble and the prospect of a major forest fire loomed. Now it was obvious a regenerative miracle had happened. Could the trees have healed themselves? I wondered.

As we approached Kelowna I was surprised to see how green the hills were. Where was all the sun-browned grass of yore? Could we be in Lancashire and not in the Okanagan?

I did know that the region had experienced record rain fall and snowpack melt. Kelowna was on flood watch when we arrived. Boating and swimming in the lakes were prohibited due to the high waters which were erasing beaches and concealing snags and other newly submerged hazards. The high waters were even challenging the clearance tolerances between Okanagan Lake and the nine-year-old William R. Bennett Bridge.

We found our hotel, the Fairmont, with relative ease. The weather was hot when we arrived. The outside temperature on our car's dash registered in the low thirties. After checking in we dined in the air-conditioned comfort of the nearby Cactus Club and retired early. Could this trip be the one on which I spotted Ogopogo, the legendary lake monster, kin to Nessie, famed in cryptobiologist and tourist lore? I asked myself as I drifted into dreamland.

The next morning we rendezvoused with Deborah Rusch from Promote Recovery of the Heart and Stroke Foundation in BC, in the reception area of the Vernon Jubilee Hospital. As Deb went to pick up lunch, Ron and I made our way to the Polson Tower for the first of the Lunch and Learn sessions.

The purpose of Deb's talk was to acquaint the health care professionals with the new program which the Heart and Stroke Foundation began offering two years ago—Living with Stroke. This program is a community-based support and educational program designed for stroke survivors and their care partners. Each program runs for six to eight weeks and is led by trained stroke survivors or professional therapists or a team of both. Unlike people who suffer from heart disease and who are usually able to return to their former lives easily, Heart and Stroke Foundation research shows that stroke survivors need and want support programs to help them cope with their recovery and with their re-integration into their communities. If this program had been offered five years ago, Ron and I might not have felt like we had been abandoned and left to flounder on our own.

Ron's subsequent talk immediately demonstrated that recovery from a stroke is a lengthy and challenging process. A stroke alters the brain, the mind and the self. The good news he shared is that the brain can heal itself and that recovery never ends. AND, he argued, if the stories of stroke survivors were taken seriously, if the anecdotal accounts of their stroke experiences were collected and collated by computer, the results would be scientifically significant. The results could teach us much about ourselves and about how the brain works. As Professor Kaku points out, the brain and the universe are our last two, equally UNKNOWN ZONES.

(Ogopogo not withstanding.)

LAKE COUNTRY

After the Lunch and Learn session at the hospital, Ron had a book signing scheduled at Bookland in downtown Vernon at 3 p.m. Deb Rusch and John, the volunteer stroke survivor who leads the Living with Stroke sessions in Vernon, also set up a table near Ron to give out information about their program. By 3:30 p.m. it was obvious to all of us that our presence was not going to draw a crowd. No doubt this was due to the intense heat. The outside temperature registered on our car's dashboard had flirted with 40 degrees Celsius. Consequently, I was prompted to quote from Stephen Leacock's piece "We Have With Us Tonight" from *My Discovery of England* in which Leacock notes that it had been his experience that audiences are very fickle creatures. They will not turn out if it's too hot, too rainy, or too cold, or if there's a hockey game in town. They often won't turn up, even if the event is free, *especially* if the event is free.

At the mention of Stephen Leacock's name, John perked up. John had had his stroke seventeen years ago and today appears to have made a full recovery (although he does confess he still has trouble reading.) However, long before his stroke, he had run a newspaper in the community of Enderby and Stephen Leacock had, for a few years, owned a cabin on a nearby lake. John had often met Leacock in the town, and, as John was able to take Leacock's disparaging quips about his paper in good humour, the two became friends. I was thrilled to learn this and to be able to claim to have met someone who had known Canada's greatest humorist. Ron, however, was downcast. By 4 p.m. he confessed that this was the first time he had ever been skunked. Not even one book sold!

Fortunately, the next day the Lunch and Learn session in the Murray Ramsden Boardroom at the Kelowna Regional Hospital was packed and the book signing at Chapters in the Orchard Park Shopping Centre later in the afternoon, a success. Local Living with Stroke facilitator and stroke survivor, Jennifer Monaghan, and many members from her groups came to keep Ron busy meeting people, swapping stroke stories, comparing notes on fatigue, trouble speaking and other stroke generated complaints.

On Wednesday Lunch and Learn was scheduled for noon in the Penticton Regional Hospital. Again, there was a good turn out of hospital staff, and Deb's and Ron's talks were well received. Then, we had to dash to Osoyoos where Ron was scheduled to read at the Bits and Bites Café in the Chase Valley Business Centre on Main Street. And here, (omitting a description of the last two of the many unnecessary detours I had taken us on throughout the day) Ron arrived only five minutes late. Again, Deb had provided provisions—coffee, tea, juice and delicious cookies from the Café—and the local stroke facilitator, Barb Roth, and many people from her group were waiting. Following Ron's talk and reading the discussion was brisk, as it usually is with stroke survivors and their caregivers. One man was upset with the local policy which requires everyone to report to the closest hospital in Oliver to be seen by a doctor who then decides whether a referral to the Penticton Hospital is necessary. This caregiver felt that this delay had worsened the effects of his wife's stroke. He was angry, for good reason. As many of us have learned, TIME **IS** BRAIN, and prompt treatment essential.

During this trip, and all the other encounters with stroke survivors that Ron and I have had on our travels, I am often shocked by the sight of stroke survivors in their wheelchairs, struggling to cope with grievous bodily harm—contorted limbs, faces swathed with drool, uncontrollable twitches or spasms in arms, legs, torsos and heads, anguished voices uttering incoherent sounds. I am always amazed by the courage these survivors show in making the effort to come to hear Ron. And I am awed by their caregivers, who have willingly shouldered the challenge of caring for these beloved family members at home.

THE KOOTENAYS

Ron and I were late leaving Osoyoos. For some reason I was unable to repack the trunk of our car in a timely fashion even though it was two cartons of books roomier. (Did I mention that I got 40 percent in mechanical aptitude in high school?) Also, I had not properly registered the fact that we were due in Nelson at noon, and I had been taking my time with our departure. Nonetheless, after tossing the bed bar in the back seat, I finally got the trunk lid shut and Ron survived the knuckle-biting ascent out of Osoyoos. (Did I mention that he is not fond of heights?) Unfortunately, we encountered two construction delays and one torrential downpour. Consequently, it was almost 1:30 p.m. when I parked on one of Nelson's main streets and got out to ask for directions to the Nelson Public Library. (Did I mention that we do not have a Smart Phone or SatNav?)

The first three people I encountered on the busy sidewalk were tourists. I changed tactics. "Are you local?" I began to ask. Eventually, after locating a local, I discovered that we were only a couple of blocks away from our destination where our host and stroke recovery facilitator, Marg Dietrich, was on duty at the library till two. After meeting librarian and author, Anne DeGrace, and unloading some books for the evening reading, Marg, Ron and I left to spend some down time at

Marg's house where Ron and I had been invited to spend the night.

Marg drove. Like most of the streets in Nelson which boast a steep slope, her driveway is almost vertical, has a sharp U-turn at the bottom and the top, and is difficult to find if you are not a local. The entrance to her driveway is also right next to the self-same steps that Steve Martin skipped down in the opening scene of *Roxanne*. I was thrilled to see them. After enjoying a cup of tea and some of Marg's home-made rhubarb coffee cake, Ron lay down on the living room couch to rest. Marg and I made a brave attempt to sit out on her deck but the storm that Ron and I had battled earlier blew in and she and I retreated to her TV room and shared a wonderful bottle of local dark ale. (Did I mention that Marg and her husband had founded the all-organic Nelson Brewing Company?)

There were six of us for dinner at Max & Irma's Kitchen. Writer Tom Wayman and author Barb Curry Mulcahy had driven in from the Slocan Valley to visit with Ron before the reading and Deborah Rusch had come to support Marg and provide informational materials about the Living with Stroke program after the reading. Meanwhile, I happily concentrated on the delicious pizza.

Attendance at the library was good. There were over thirty people present even though a local author, whose mystery novel had just won a prize in Europe, was also appearing at a nearby venue.

Ron's reading was excellent. The audience asked lots of questions. And my long-time friend, Suzanne, and I even had a chance to visit.

Last year Suzanne suffered a stroke, and she is now a member of Marg Dietrich's Living with Stroke group. Marg tailors her program to individual needs, so I'm confident Suzanne will benefit from Marg's insights.

LOCAL and LOCO

On Friday, June 2 Ron and I left Nelson rather earlier than we had planned to. Word of Ron's tour had spread and, consequently, he had received an invitation to talk at the Kootenay Boundary Regional Hospital in Trail. En route we passed BC's largest lead-zinc smelter. It would have been impossible to miss the giant, silver, tubular structure which dwarfs the buildings in town. By following the green H hospital signs, we found our way to our destination without any problems, and, at 1 p.m., Ron spoke to a gathering of about twenty hospital staff in the comfortable setting of the Board Room. As usual his audience was full of questions and by 2:30 we were ready for a chocolate dipped soft ice cream cone from the Dairy Queen we had spotted in the centre of town.

After cooling off, we needed directions to Highway 3 and the road to Creston. At one of the therapist's suggestions, we had decided to head for the new Ramada Inn there. Drawing on my recent experiences in Nelson, I approached a silver-haired lady in the parking lot who was heading for her truck.

"Excuse me," I said. "Are you local?"

"Local AND loco," she replied.

"Excellent. Is this the road to Creston?" I asked pointing to the road heading east.

"The very one," she said. "Just follow it up the hill and keep on going."

At the Kootenay Pass Summit, we slowed down

for a family of Bighorn Mountain Sheep grazing by the side of the highway. After a short but steep descent we entered the valley in which the town of Creston is sited. In my opinion, this is one of the most beautiful places in British Columbia and during our three day stay in Creston we seriously considered what it would be like to live there.

Features to recommend Creston:

1. An intact, original, living town centre with free parking, lots of parking spots for the disabled, lots of benches and well-kept flower plantings.
2. No big box stores.
3. Two picturesque grain elevators.
4. An abundance of orchards and farms.
5. A few kilometres' drive away from the southern tip of Kootenay Lake.
6. A Wildlife Interpretive Centre near a wetland on the edge of town.
7. Tim's Fish and Chips where the staff wear T-shirts sporting "Oh my Cod!" and "Just for the Halibut," and the portions are double what you expect.
8. A wonderful, refurbished recreation complex, with a new swimming pool which has wheelchair access for the disabled.

And, most important, we got lots of much needed REST in C-rest-on.

STROKE MONTH SAGA, continued: CALGARY, Alberta

On Monday, June 5th Ron and I proceeded east on #3, the Crowsnest Highway. The highway takes its name from the Crowsnest Pass in the Rockies where the road crosses the Continental Divide between BC and Alberta.

However, it is not my intention to dwell on descriptions of the flora and fauna or geological phenomena such as the Frank Slide. Nor will I comment on my *faux pas* in consulting a map of BC and Alberta published in 1998 when planning our route to Calgary along Highway #22. Nor will I describe the fits of frustrated frenzy the author of *The Defiant Mind* threw when he realized that he was headed back to the Rocky Mountains and not to Calgary. Also, I will omit any mention of the difficulties one is likely to encounter when asking for directions at gas stations in Calgary. Suffice it to say that I did not encounter a local, at least not a local whose first language was English and who knew the city like a chuckwagon driver would know the track at the Calgary Stampede. I shall also refrain from describing the logistics of navigating our way to our hotel—my cousin Cheryl being away on a hiking tour in the bucolic Tyrolean Alps. Instead, I shall simply remain grateful that somehow we found our way to the hotel, marriage in tatters but luggage intact, and happy in the knowledge that it was only 4 p.m.;

that Ron did not have to be at the reading at Shelf Life Books until seven; that Noreen Kamal and her husband were picking us up at the hotel at 6:30 p.m.; and that I would not have to drive.

In recognition of June as Stroke Awareness Month, the event at the bookstore had a unique format. Ron's reading was complemented by Dr. Noreen Kamal, a Researcher and Adjunct Assistant Professor at the University of Calgary, the engineer who is responsible for implementing the world-leading stroke treatment now available throughout Alberta; and by neurologist, Dr. Amy Yu, who graciously stepped in on short notice for Dr. Michael Hill who had been called away to Hamilton and Toronto. The women were there to comment on stroke and to answer questions from the audience. The answers they gave were extremely enlightening, even more so because their Department of Clinical Neurosciences at the University of Calgary is world renowned. Dr. Hill and his team led the international research and randomised trials for endovascular thrombectomy for large vessel blockages in ischemic strokes.

Using this procedure, a person suffering from a clot in the brain has a tube inserted into a blood vessel in their groin which can then be sent all the way up into the brain where a stent is released into the blood clot. Then the stent and the clot can be pulled back down the tube and out the blood vessel in the groin.

Doctors Kamal and Yu are intimately familiar

with all aspects of stroke treatment and understand how and when endovascular thrombectomy may be applicable and how effective the treatment can be in substantially reducing the disabilities which typically result from ischemic strokes. As one of the caregivers in the audience, I was pleased to hear about a treatment that would lead to less debilitating outcomes. I think all of us rejoiced in this news.

HEART and STROKE

The next day, Ron and I drove to the Heart and Stroke offices in Calgary. Just to set your minds at ease, let me assure you that I had first consulted Google Maps in the hotel business area and had directions to our destination printed out. In addition, I had charted the route on my 2017 map of the city of Calgary. The distance was comparatively short and my call to Kristine Skogg, CEO Donna Hasting's assistant, earlier in the morning had ensured that we would be able to unload the books Donna had ordered for each of her managers in the back alley behind the red brick building which houses the Heart and Stroke offices. All went as planned. Ron and I even got an escort to the parking lot where our Handicap Parking Permit was immediately put to good use.

Ron and I then had the privilege of meeting and talking to Lou and Frank Nieboer. The Nieboers have been married for fifty years, an admirable record made even more remarkable given that Lou had a serious stroke forty years ago when she was just thirty-four. Today she still bears the effects of her brain attack, although she insists on walking without a cane; but, I noted, she does lean on Frank's arm.

I was taken aback when she said the capacity she misses the most, though, is her biting wit. Somehow her cutting repartee is still missing in action, but, like every other ability she has fought to regain, she is determined to rediscover it as well.

Obviously the Nieboers have been a terrific team. Frank is the namesake and recipient of the first "Heart & Stroke—Heart of Gold Volunteer Award" for exemplary long-time volunteering as Chair of the Alberta Board, member of the Heart and Stroke Foundation of Canada Board, founder of the Alberta Stroke Recovery Association and numerous other contributions. Both Frank and Lou have worked tirelessly to increase awareness and promote stroke recovery in Alberta and across Canada. Their devotion to each other and their work is inspirational.

After lunch Ron opened his presentation by reading the passage from *The Defiant Mind* which describes his encounter with a fellow stroke survivor after a therapy session. Although the passage is long, I think it's worth quoting parts of it here, for it (and a couple of other passages which Ron read) generated a lot of insightful questions and discussion about what constitutes effective therapy for stroke survivors. The feedback from Ron's presentation was certainly positive with fifteen out of seventeen of the Heart and Stroke Managers rating it the highlight of their Learning and Development Day.

> I noticed a woman who had been admitted to the rehab unit around the same time as I was, sitting on one of the blue-matted exercise benches. The gym had emptied and was quiet, the way a museum can get near closing.... The woman's head was downcast and

her posture was one of total defeat. Before I had my stroke I probably would have turned away, quietly, and left the room.... She was slumped over as if she wanted to sink through the floor. I sat down beside her and rested my elbows on my knees. This was difficult because my right arm still wouldn't bend the way it was supposed to and still caused me considerable pain....

For over a minute we just sat there staring at our feet, waiting, waiting as you do for the tide to come in or for the sun to set, waiting for the right moment to speak. Everything about the way she held herself worried me.

... Then I noticed tears running down her cheeks.

She was pale and her face was carved into the sort of chunks you sometimes see in a Francis Bacon or Picasso portrait. She had a modest beauty, one I suspect she had been unaware of or unconcerned about throughout her life.... She had two sons and a husband who visited her daily. She was one of the lucky ones. Doted on, from what I could tell....

"You okay?" I asked.

A foolish question, but I knew I needed to get her to talk.

"Yes."

She gave me a quick glance.

"No."

Now she studied me. Her grey eyes looked hollowed out and seemed to have sunk back into her skull over the past few weeks....

"You're doing so well," she said. "I've been watching you."

She tried to smile, but the effort it took was too great, and her lips collapsed back into a grim line....

"It's so difficult," she said. "I can't do what you do, and we've been in here about the same length of time."...

"It's impossible for you to see how you're doing. You can't see yourself," I insisted. "You have to be convinced that you're making progress. Then you will," I said.

I understood this despair. I had gone through this conversation with myself many times. Only other stroke survivors knew what you were going through, but there just wasn't a vocabulary adequate to describe the ebb and flow of emotions....

"I've tried so hard. I do everything they ask of me. But I still need the wheelchair."

"Every stroke is different," I said, repeating the one tired answer that remains a constant in stroke dialogues, the one response which she didn't want to hear from me, not from someone who was actually living inside a stroke....

"It takes time," I said, fumbling over my words ... "so much time for all of us. You just can't give up."

"Before the stroke I had two heart attacks," she said. "Compared to this they were a piece of cake."

Then a sad look seeped back into her eyes.

"I thought it would be the same. After both heart attacks I was back on my feet within a month or two. Not with this, though. I can't see a way out."

As if sensing danger, she visibly recoiled. Like a snail, withdrawing into its shell. She gave me her hand which was cold and bony. Then I felt her body shiver and stiffen, her lungs fill, her eyes stare resolutely into mine, and it was then that I knew that, despite her apparent despair, she would never give up. She was one of those people who in the face of terror find the strength to be brave.

"I just have to accept the fact that I'll never be the same. I'll never be the same person I was," she said. "Part of me has died."

She paused to try to take in fully what it was she had just admitted to herself.

"And I must remind myself that I can't do what you do," she added. "As you say, we're all different. Our brains are different." (pp. 44–47)

After a short break Kate Chidester made a presentation on "Fueling the Brightest Research" and Dr. Hank Duff spoke about "Why Heart and Stroke Research is So Important." He talked about the seminal effect the research grants he and some of his colleagues had received from the Heart and Stroke Foundation early in their careers. This funding had encouraged the establishment of a gifted team of heart researchers and specialists in Calgary. The freedom that these scientists were given in their research allowed for the development of a meritocracy, which, through self-selection made significant and serendipitous discoveries.

Calgary, it seems, is doubly blessed with world-class people in BOTH heart and stroke.

In answer to a question about whether specific areas for research funding should be identified Dr. Duff paused to consider his answer.

"No," he finally replied. "As in all areas of human endeavour, people learn and progress by making mistakes and we must always allow researchers the freedom to fail and thereby to learn."

In my own small way, I understood what he was saying. Caregivers need to feel the freedom to fail as well because we all will fail in some small way whether over negotiations about meals, dress, exercise, rest, medications, entertainment or whatever care is needed at any particular moment. A signal will be missed, and an inexplicable tension will enter the relationship. It's unavoidable.

Dr. Duff's invitation to speak at the meeting had also been part of a ruse to get him to attend. Unbeknownst to him, he was going to be presented with the "Frank Nieboer—Heart & Stroke Heart of Gold Award" by Frank himself. Dr. Duff is the third recipient of this esteemed award since its inception in 2007.

ENTERING the SQUARED CIRCLE

At the Stroke Recovery Association of Calgary's annual convention at the Coombs Theatre in the Foothills Medical Centre in Calgary on Saturday, June 10th Ron was "bottom of the card." Thanks to the advice of locals, and thanks to the ride provided by Donna Hastings, who picked Ron and me up at the hotel and let us off at the front door of the hospital, I did not have to navigate, drive or park and we arrived with ample time to spare. The Foothills Medical Centre was undergoing massive re-construction and parking was a nightmare, particularly for people with disabilities. Some people I spoke to even questioned the wisdom of choosing the Coombs Theatre, the SRAC's usual venue, for this year's convention. Possibly a hockey rink might have been a better choice? suggested some.

By 10 a.m. Ron had made his way down the stairs to the podium in the large lecture room and was seated at a table behind a microphone. Vicky Jones, the Association's President, made her opening remarks, introduced Ron and the convention was officially under way. Ron's audience was half the size of previous years. Given the parking situation, only 100 people were in the audience. 200 people were the norm, a number corroborated by the generous amount of food later provided at lunch.

For the first time on the trip I was unable to hear Ron's presentation. I was outside the theatre in the lobby seated behind a table displaying bookmarks and copies of *The Defiant Mind*. This table was next to one of two entrances to the theatre. The only time I was able to catch a peek inside was when late arrivals opened the doors to let themselves in. Occasionally I would hear the sounds of rippling laughter, and at 10:45 a.m. it was impossible to miss the sirens and the announcement that FIRE ALARM TESTING IS NOW COMPLETE.

But Ron was not the main event. The guest speaker with "top billing" was Bret "The Hit Man" Hart, famous in the international world of professional wrestling. He was due up on the SRAC's card at 1 p.m., after lunch. Hart is also known as "King of the Ring" or "Master of the Squared Circle." He has held the World Wrestling title seven times and numerous other championships over a span of five decades from the 1970s to the 2010s. The son of a famous Calgary wrestling dynasty, he is well-known locally for his wrestling exploits and for his support and endorsement of the Calgary Hitmen, who play in the Central Division of the Western Hockey League.

What is not so well known is that Bret Hart suffered a stroke in 2002. Although he was completely paralyzed on his left side for a time, he was able to return to the ring in 2003 after recovering his ability to bench press 300 pounds. Yet he still suffers from the emotional after-effects of his stroke. The double doors to the lobby were twice thrown open when a gentleman from the audience came out and grabbed a handful of napkins left over from lunch to give to Hart to help him stem the tears that fell non-stop throughout his address. Ron attended and confirmed that Hart had given a *heart*-felt and moving speech.

For me, the most emotional part of the day came later in the afternoon when Ron and I met the husband of a woman who was a patient on the stroke ward in the hospital. Word of all the tasty treats, available FOR FREE in the lobby of the Coombs Theatre, had spread to the stroke ward after a couple of the nurses there had come down to fill up trays to take upstairs for staff, family and patients. The husband had arrived in the Theatre to partake of the food. He appeared to be in his late forties and his wife was probably close to the same age. Her stroke had hit a few weeks earlier, a stroke which had left her "locked in." Even at one of the world's foremost stroke treatment centres some strokes cannot be helped and they continue to take life-shattering tolls.

After her stroke, the only parts of her body this woman was able to move were her eyes. With the help of a computer and her eyes she was able to communicate some of her needs and wants to her husband and to the therapists who daily move her legs and arms to keep her large muscle systems active. Her husband was hopeful that new discoveries in mind-machine interface (MMI) might soon be available to help his wife, particularly as her neurologist was about to head to Geneva for an international conference where the most up-to-date findings in this field would be shared.

All stroke stories are emotionally powerful, but I found this gentleman's account of his wife's stroke one of the most moving I had listened to. It reminded me, once again, of *The Diving Bell and the Butterfly* by Jean-Dominique Bauby. After his paralyzing stroke, Bauby dictated his memoir by blinking his left eyelid (his right was sewn shut) in response to the correct letter pointed to by a speech therapist using a French language frequency-ordered alphabet. The composition took several months of four-hour daily sessions. Bauby would compose and memorize a passage during the night and dictate his text the following day. On March 6, 1997 his book was published. The author died two days later.

We celebrate sporting accomplishments, quite rightly, but seldom acknowledge personal, life-changing marvels.

There are heroes.

By 3 p.m. Ron and I were ready to leave. Thanks to a ride from Bev Culham, Manager of Health Promotion for the Heart and Stroke Foundation, we were able to arrive safe and dry at the hotel where our luggage was waiting for us at reception. Once behind the wheel of our trusty Toyota, luggage intact, I was able to navigate the twists and turns of the service road with all the *savoir faire* of a native Calgarian. Quickly out of the maze we found ourselves on Trans-Canada Number One, heading west. Even though we were late for a rendezvous in Canmore, with Dianne and Ron Deans, I drove slowly through the heavy traffic heading for the Rockies—through the torrents of a downpour, known by locals as *The June Monsoon*—happy in the knowledge that our Stroke Month Saga was nearly over. We were heading WEST at last and I revelled in the promise that we would be HOME, SOON.

<u>THE DEFIANT MIND</u> goes INTERNATIONAL

Reader's Digest International published a fifteen-page excerpt based on Ron's book in their June 2018 issue. The international edition reaches six million readers in fourteen countries. According to Thomas Dobrowski, *Reader's Digest's* Global Rights Manager, the publication distributes in English in the UK, Australia, India and Canada; and has translated editions in Spanish, French, Portuguese, Dutch, Slovenian, Chinese, Finnish, Swedish, and Norwegian. (Online, Ron found an issue published in Urdu, and he's heard murmurs that it might have been published in Turkish.)

Reader's Digest went on to publish the excerpt from Ron's book in their American and Canadian editions, the latter appearing in early 2020.

Our adventures with *The Defiant Mind* or Ron's stroke have not stopped. We continue to visit stroke recovery groups. We continue to meet people leading inspiring lives. We still have books and will travel. Yet a major change occurred in our lives in the fall of 2017. We sold our dream house and moved into a townhouse close by.

One stage of our lives had ended.

Another had begun.

PART THREE
Mind and Matter
Body and Soul

My initial response to Ron's unexpected brain attack was shock and fear. Followed by denial. Everything I have experienced since has taught me what a stroke can do to the human spirit, body and soul, and what it means to be a caregiver. On reflection, I have come to understand that caregiving lives in every cell of our being.

Any tragic, life-altering event causes the people affected to face their own mortality. Daily we live as if we were immortal, but at any moment, we can discover how tenuous our hold on life is. We can be diagnosed with cancer, suffer a heart attack or a stroke, be hit by a car, become the parent of a severely disabled child, or the sole support of a spouse, a sibling, an elderly parent or even a friend.

The cold tingle of death trips up and down our spines.

At some point the perennial questions of life, death, justice and meaning inevitably surface.

During the nine years that I have been a caregiver I have had much time to ponder these age-old riddles. Indeed, I have been contemplating them since I was a child. What I do know is that mind and matter, body and soul are linked.

Mens sana in corpore sono. A healthy mind in a healthy body.

Anima sana in corpore sono. A healthy soul in a healthy body.

The state of the mind influences the body, and the health of the body influences the mind. In this final part of the book, I have loosely traced the evolution of my thoughts about what being a caregiver means and suggested why it is imperative that we all become caregivers. I hope these meanderings will also help to demonstrate the importance of creating a *companionable* state of mind and give some clues as to how to achieve it. For the first person that a caregiver must care for is their self. S/he must be his or her own best friend.

CHAPTER ONE

Giving

For many years I resisted calling myself a caregiver. I consciously rejected the term, although initially I never thought to examine the source of my aversion. I now suspect that being as committed as I was to *full recovery,* I expected my world would some day soon return to normal, that Ron would heal completely, and I would no longer be a caregiver. It was a temporary condition only. At some future point I would return simply to being Ron's wife, Nicole and Owen's mother, Iain and Jen's mother-in-law, and Flora's grandmother. (I had yet to become Lochlan and Anja's grandmother.) All these identities I readily embraced. Admitting to being a *caregiver* meant facing up to a reality I wasn't prepared to accept. A reality that meant Ron would be permanently handicapped and in continual need of my assistance.

On the wall of our dining room in our dream house we had hung a framed broadside of a poem by Alberto Rios. Alberto gave the poem to Ron in 2005 when Ron held the inaugural Fulbright Chair in Creative Writing at Arizona State University. In the years after Ron's stroke I often stopped to read and re-read it:

When Giving Is All We Have

One river gives
Its journey to the next.

We give because someone gave to us.
We give because nobody gave to us.

We give because giving has changed us.
We give because giving could have changed us.

We have been better for it,
We have been wounded by it—

Giving has many faces: It is loud and quiet,
Big and small, diamond and wood nails.

The story is old, the plot is worn,
But we read the book, anyway, again and again:

Giving is, first and every time, hand to hand,
Mine to yours, yours to mine.

You gave me blue and I gave you yellow.
Together we are green. You gave me

What you did not have and I gave you
What I had to give—together, we made

Something greater from the difference.

I also rebelled against the reductionism the term *caregiver* implied. It suggested to me that I now belonged to the legion of people who were no longer masters of their own destiny but slaves to the needs of others. Somehow identifying as a caregiver felt wrong to me. It said to me that the scope of my life had contracted. Whereas, in many ways, it had grown immeasurably.

Perhaps I also believed the word oversimplified Ron's and my new situation. If I were a care-*giver* did that make Ron a care-*taker*? Weren't we more like comrades in arms? The mutuality of Alberto's poem felt more accurate to me. Often, Ron and I put on brave faces for each other. Ron didn't want to complain about his new afflictions for fear of being a burden while I felt I couldn't complain about my situation because I wasn't the one who was disabled.

Another word that I initially had trouble with was remembering to say stroke *survivor* rather than stroke *victim*. Although *victim* still has the ring of truth for me, I agree that *survivor* is the more empowering word.

In these days of political correctness and over-sensitivity to the role words have in conditioning our thinking, in our eagerness not to upset or offend, I fear that many words and human experiences have been robbed of their power. Another expression I do not like is *loved ones*. The more I hear it the less I like it. *Loved ones* is so general a term that it feels almost meaningless to me. I prefer the specificity of the words family and friends, lover, husband, wife, mother, father, sister, brother, son, daughter and so forth. I can hate my mother but be devastated when she dies. Every relationship that we have with another human being is always complex, multifaceted and evolving.

I also dislike the use of the word *pass* instead of *die*. Saying *s/he passed* instead of *s/he died* is a euphemism of the first order. I feel it robs us of the dignity of our mortality and suggests that we somehow slip away unnoticed into murky shadows. S/he was just passing by. S/he didn't like the hand s/he was dealt so s/he passed.

No "bloody unbowed heads" here.
No "death shall have no dominion."
Caregiving.
A reality with limits which chaffed.

As a student of the *I Ching*, the ancient Chinese *Book of Changes*, I know well enough that all "human life is conditioned and un-free." Yet I also appreciate that the ancient Greeks believed the Gods were secretly jealous of humans, whose mortality made each person unique, and, in bravely facing their inevitable fate, each human being could potentially turn into a hero or a heroine.

Like stroke survivors seen through the lens of *The Hero with a Thousand Faces*, or like the soldiers who have been maimed and disabled by war, and whose courage is celebrated in Prince Harry's Invictus Games, I tried to identify with the sentiment expressed in William Ernest Henley's poem:

Out of the night that covers me,
Black as the Pit from pole to pole,
I thank whatever gods may be
For my unconquerable soul.

In the fell clutch of circumstance
I have not winced nor cried aloud.
Under the bludgeonings of chance
My head is bloody, but unbowed.

Beyond this place of wrath and tears
Looms but the Horror of the shade,
And yet the menace of the years
Finds, and shall find me unafraid.

It matters not how strait the gate,
How charged with punishments the scroll,
I am the master of my fate:
I am the captain of my soul.

At the core of our beings, I believe that we need to know our lives are meaningful. In the knowledge of our certain death, we need to feel that the space between our beginning and our ending is important. We want to know that what we do matters. To ourselves, to our families, to our communities, and ultimately, to the Earth, herself. That is why the Journey of the Hero resonates. And why we tell heroic stories again and again and again. We need to believe that, despite all the suffering and torment being human brings, we can triumph after all.

As Anthony Storr suggests in his book, *Solitude: A Return to the Self*, "Confidence that one is of value and significance as a unique individual is one of the most precious possessions one can have." In a world where secularism and consumerism are desecrating the globe this confidence becomes ever harder to discover. We no longer count for being good; we are counted by the amount of goods we own. Our status is dependent on the kind of car we drive, the size of our houses, the designer labels we wear, the number of likes we get on Facebook.

As a teenager I attended the Sunday morning classes for teenagers which were held in the basement of the Kamloops United Church at 421 St. Paul Street in the early sixties. These sleepy sessions were led by a local doctor whose name I no longer remember. I do remember that he generally wore a well-worn tweed jacket, a sweater vest and dark brown corduroy pants. He sat beside a metal table at the front of the basement meeting room smoking his pipe while he attempted to engage us in philosophical questions such as:

Why are human beings the only creatures on Earth who have souls?

Why do dogs, for example, not have souls?

The good doctor's questions did not produce the spirited theological debate he desired but they certainly started me thinking. As far as I could tell my affectionate, intelligent dog, Twinkle, possessed all the animate features that I had, except perhaps for language. But even that was questionable, for each day when I got home from school and asked Twink what she had done while I was away, she would reply with delightfully modulated, throaty sounds. And we would proceed to converse in an expressive, pre-verbal language.

How could I be saved and Twinkle not?

At the Thursday evening convocation class for teens the Minister was in charge. He was a straight shooter. No debates wanted here. Just absolute faith in the play book. No doubt he had honed this attitude during his professional football career. To be a member of the United Church it was necessary to accept that "all have sinned and fall short of the glory of God" (Romans 3:23). Sinful people need absolution, mercy and forgiveness. Something only the divine can give. In order to be saved I would have to believe that Jesus Christ was willing and able to save me. I would have to swear that Jesus was my Lord and Saviour.

To further complicate matters, I had read a little Plato and been intrigued by Socrates' discussions with his students about what constituted the good life and their conversations about how to achieve it.

Happily, I was university bound. Convocation could wait. At university, in the hallowed halls of learning, I would find myself in the company of the *wise* who would not only know what the good life was, but they would also know how to achieve it. Imagine my disappointment when I found myself in courses such as "Statistics for the Behavioural Sciences." Perhaps the term *political science* should have warned me off?

Thankfully I chanced upon Religious Studies and discovered that here goodness and the good life were talked about and I discovered they could mean very different things to people in diverse cultures and civilizations. For example, Hinduism views human beings as ignorant rather than as sinful. Therefore, it is possible, say Hindus, for people to liberate themselves with knowledge. By their own thoughts and actions, it is possible for people to rid themselves of their ignorance of their ultimate nature by replacing it with the knowledge of their true self.

I much preferred to think of myself as ignorant rather than sinful. Like John Milton in *Paradise Lost* I intuitively felt that "The mind is in its own place and in itself can make a Heaven of Hell, a Hell of Heaven."

One might even call the mind *defiant*.

CHAPTER TWO

Suffering

Like Hinduism, Buddhism asserts that human beings are ignorant of the true nature of mind and matter. But unlike Hindus or Christians, Buddhists do not believe in a soul, or a god. Where Hindus find an ultimate essence which permeates all being, Buddhists see nothing or non-being. Extinction of the self is the way to *nirvana*.

The Buddha was a pragmatist. He declared that debates about the nature of ultimate reality weren't helpful. His teachings, known as the Four Noble Truths, were originally formulated like an ancient Indian medical diagnosis. Identify the problem. Isolate the cause. Describe the cure. Prescribe the remedy.

1. To live a human life, he said, is to suffer. The essence of life is suffering.
2. The cause of this suffering is the transitory nature of mind and matter. Everything is in constant flux and change. The only thing that is permanent is change. Everything that comes into being inevitably ceases to be.
3. Humans constantly cling to things, to situations, to people—all of which will cease to be. When this happens, they suffer. Therefore, the cure for suffering is to stop clinging.

4. The way to effect this cure is to embrace the Holy Eightfold Path—right views, right intentions, right speech, right conduct, right livelihood, right effort, right mindfulness and right concentration.

When a member of your family becomes ill or disabled, you fear for them.
You fear for yourself.
You get angry.
You despair.
You worry.
In short, you suffer.

Two books I found particularly helpful when my stress levels were at their highest were Thich Nhat Hanh's *No Death, No Fear* and *The Miracle of Mindfulness*. The number of books this Buddhist monk has penned is legion. Yet the message at the heart of most of them is essentially the same: the way to free yourself from fear, anger, despair, worry and suffering is to stay focused on the present moment. The past is gone forever. The future hasn't arrived yet, and we have no idea what it will bring. The only place where we exist is in the present moment. So, says Hanh, give the present moment your full attention, all the time.

When you are washing the dishes be aware of the temperature of the water, the bubbles that the soap produces. Note the shine on the clean dishes. See how the light reflects and flashes in your eye. Smell the aroma of the soap. Bring your full attention to the task. Deepen your breath. Don't rush.

When you walk, sit, move, talk, breathe, smile, pray or drink a cup of tea be grateful for the present moment. When you do this your cares dissolve and happiness is possible, for happiness happens when suffering ceases.

After Ron's stroke, I found concentrating on the present and stopping my worries about the future particularly helpful. The more I learned how to control my thoughts and ignore the future, the more worry I gave up and let go. The more worry I gave up, the more space I created for unexpected events to occur.

People stepped in and filled voids.

Help arrived, without my consciously asking for it or willing it, at the precise moments I needed it.

The practice of controlling thoughts is not easy. Ask anyone who has attempted to meditate. Thoughts are like wild horses. They skittishly gallop off in all directions. Like Stephen Leacock's man who mounts his horse and rides off in all directions at once. A few attempts to sit quietly and concentrate on your breathing should be enough to convince you that it is your thoughts that control you and not you who control them. The way to control your thoughts, say Hindus and Buddhists, is to control your breath. In fact, they even measure a life span by the number of breaths taken and not by the number of years lived. If you want to live longer deepen your breath.

Most of the time our thoughts bounce from one sense object to another, projecting into the future one moment, and then pivoting and recalling the past the next. Writers like James Joyce and Virginia Wolf brilliantly illustrate this constant thrum of the mind in their novels using a technique called *stream of consciousness*.

In his book, *Flow: The Psychology of Optimal Experience,* psychologist Mihaly Csikzentmihalyi suggests that consciousness is the result of complex biological processes in our nervous systems determined by instructions contained in the protein molecules of our chromosomes. Yet, he argues, consciousness is not solely determined by its biological programming. It can also be self-directed. It is possible to change your state of mind, to make yourself happy or miserable, simply by changing the contents of your thoughts. Seemingly hopeless situations can be transformed into obstacles to be overcome. The ability to do this is a trait we justly admire. It leads, not only to success in life, but to the enjoyment of life as well.

Flow is the state of mind which occurs when a person is totally absorbed in a challenging and worthwhile task. It is a state like that which others have described as "being in the zone." A state when a golfer's putts continually find the hole. When all a basketball player's shots fall. When ideas for a book continually pop into a writer's mind. A state when a seamstress or a cook or a welder is wholly engaged with their creation. A state where solutions to problems present themselves, seemingly out of nowhere. This often happens when the rational conscious mind is relaxed; when a person is in one of the 3 B's—the bed, the bus or the bath. A state in which the Zen archer is thinking about "nothing," a state in which s/he has all her skill. *Flow* is what Diane Ackerman describes as *deep play*—an activity engaged in by all mammals, where learning, discovery and skills are honed. When we are doing what we love.

Unfortunately *flow* states are fleeting. It seems that we are not often *in the zone*. It is a condition that needs to be sought. Our environment needs to be conducive for *flow* to occur. As caregivers we need to find out what activities engage us in *deep play*. We need to make time for them even when our circumstances dramatically change. One lady I met at one of Ron's readings said that after her husband's stroke he became extremely angry. So much so, that it became no longer possible for her to live with him. Their solution: to live side by side, in separate apartments.

Things change, but if you practice concentrating on the present moment and deepen your breath, the changes will cause you much less worry and stress. You will find yourself *playing* more often.

Too often caregivers can get caught in patterns of thinking which lead them into negative emotional and intellectual feedback loops. In *Surviving Stroke* Dr. Helen Kennerley devotes an entire chapter to cognitive behavioural therapy (CBT), which teaches people strategies for keeping fear, anger, grief and hopelessness at bay. Learning new ways of coping can help caregivers keep their situations in perspective and help them to better manage their own problems,

In the early years after Ron's stroke, another helpful concept that I drew on from my university studies was the Hindu ideal of the Four Stages of Life. According to time honoured tradition, the first stage of life (for upper caste males) was that of the chaste student. (Please note, I never let gender distinctions dissuade me from taking profound advice to heart.) It was customary for a young man to move into the home of a master with whom he would study the Vedas, the ancient Sanskrit holy scriptures and their six ancillary studies: phonetics, phonology and pronunciation; prosody, the study of poetic meters; grammar; etymology; ritual instructions; and auspicious time keeping, astrology and astronomy. These six *limbs* were aids to the proper understanding of the Vedas.

When the student had completed his studies, he would marry and establish his own household. During the second stage of life, the householder phase, he was expected to take on all the social responsibilities of this station—care for an extended family, raise children, earn a living, pay taxes—in short, he was to live in the world fully, enjoying all its sensual and aesthetic pleasures, as well as fulfilling all its responsibilities. But this stage should not last a lifetime.

Once a man sees his first grandchild, he knows that it is now time for him to withdraw from the cares and rewards of the world. It is time for him to hand over all his worldly responsibilities to the next generation and to assist in an advisory capacity only. It is time for him to retire to the forest and enter the third stage of life, that of the forest-dweller. When he retires to the forest, he may take his wife with him or leave her for her sons to care for. In the forest, he lives simply, eats light food, wears unadorned clothes. He returns to the studies of his youth but, during the third stage of life, his goal is not simply learning and rote memorization. Armed with the wisdom, knowledge and maturity gained from his life in the world, he is now expected to realize for himself the truth of his student studies. Ideally, he will experience the truth that *tat tvam asi*. That *thou art that*. That his true self is identical with ultimate reality. That *Atman* is *Brahman*. That the divine spark in man is identical with God.

While I was outside *forest-bathing*, living the much simpler lifestyle that Ron's stroke had imposed, I imagined myself to be a forest-dweller. I concentrated on my raking, deeply breathing in the smell of the cedar and fir trees, listening to the crackle of arbutus leaves, delighting in the antics of squirrels, contemplating the flight of eagles and turkey vultures, treasuring the croak of tree frogs, spooking the deer who were intent on eating my flowers.

As the years went by, one change became increasingly apparent. While the trees were expanding, I was literally shrinking. I am now an inch and a half shorter than I used to be. When I turned seventy, I appreciated that the trees were going to continue to grow up, while I was going to continue to grow down. It was time to sell our dream house and downsize. I was ready for the fourth stage of life.

In India this stage of life is called the stage of re-nunciation. This is the final phase of life where *sannyasins* (male) and *sannyasinis* (female) renounce their identities, their families and their homes and become wandering mendicants. They completely detach them-selves from their former lives, not caring whether they live or whether they die. They become *yatrasayamgriha rishis*. Wherever (*yatra*) they find themselves at night, that is where they make their (*sayam*) home (*griha*). Obviously, this is easier to do in India where, apart from the monsoon season, the climate is much kinder to homeless wanderers than Canada's. Also, household-ers in India are happy to fill mendicants' begging bowls with food. Not a common practice here.

The fourth stage Ron and I opted for was to sell our dream house and move into a townhouse. Whether or not we will discover further stages past this one, I do not know. We are westerners, after all, and much at-tached to our creature comforts. But I do know one thing for certain—I am not going to ruin the present by worrying about the future.

Recently I discovered the Well Spouse Association website and learned that there are clearly defined stages in caregiving, too, although the boundaries can blur. It is always possible to take a couple of steps forward and then fall back. According to the featured article by

Marty Beilin entitled *The Caregiver Journey: Pathways to an Authentic and Fulfilling life* the first stage is the Heroic Stage. In this stage optimism often abounds, as the well spouse determines to do everything they can to help the ill spouse heal. Certainly, I willingly embraced getting Ron out of the hospital and home to my care as soon as possible. Full recovery was my goal. Yet, when the first anniversary of Ron's stroke arrived, we were both depressed by the glacial progress he was making, despite our best efforts.

Eventually I began to realize that stroke recovery was going to be a long-term proposition. Stage Two—Ambivalence—had arrived. According to Beilin this is the time when caregivers start to experience internal conflicts, physical exhaustion, financial worries, and even clinical depressions—the time when my mantra unconsciously became *I Need a Break. I Need a Break. I Need a Break.*

Stage Three, the New Normal, happens when the caregiver has come to terms with his or her long-term situation and has found new ways of coping. This may include placing the ill spouse in a nursing home, finding adult day care, and for some, it may even include divorce.

The first time I heard the term "the new normal" was when Tina, our Rehab Social Worker, used it, when Ron was only two months post-stroke. After we told Tina that we didn't need any of the financial assistance programs that she could offer us then, and that we seemed to be coping OK, she suggested that we had reached the new normal. In fact, our lives were anything but normal as we both grappled with our dramatically altered condition. Emotionally we were fragile, and I know I was still somewhat in shock. I believe I was even in denial.

At first Ron and I were just struggling to cope. That we managed as well as we did was due to the support of family and friends, and people from our larger community. Ultimately the main reason why we have reached a stage which I would now agree is our new normal, is because we have been able to build a bridge between our pre-stroke selves and our post-stroke selves. While Ron's stroke left him physically and emotionally challenged, his cognitive functions and his relationships to the language, while changed, were not impaired. As I said earlier: he did not suffer with aphasia; he continued to be able to say what he meant; his words made sense, even if his pronunciation was sometimes garbled; he could communicate with friends via the internet; he was able to edit the works of others; and he could still write his stroke memoir. Each afternoon he would read aloud the new sections he had written that morning, while I sat, listened and commented on what I had just heard. We continued to share our passion for literature. We were able to live what the Well Spouse folks call authentic lives, continuing to do what we had always loved.

I cannot emphasize enough the importance of retaining a connection between a person's pre-stroke self and their post-stroke self. As Dr. Helen Kennerly states:

Udo's first consultant on the Stroke Unit was someone who knew him professionally, and she called him "Professor" from the outset, a thoughtful gesture that gave him dignity and elevated him from disabled patient to the person he was. As we were to come to appreciate more and more, it is so important not to lose sight of the person and the therapeutic power of dignity. (*Surviving Stroke,* p. 23)

CHAPTER THREE

Duty

When I was a child, around the age of eight or nine, I used to spend some time pondering the question: *Why was I who I was?*

Why was I born to my parents? And not to my friend Marion's, for example?

Why was I born at this time? And not in the time of Queen Elizabeth the First?

Why was I born here? And not there?

These questions usually surfaced during late sunlit summer evenings when I knelt by the wooden sash of my window in the upstairs bedroom I shared with my younger brother. I remember having my chin resting in my hands, my elbows on the window ledge, as I knelt in my pink cotton nightgown and looked out on our green lawn and longed to be outside playing. Billy, as I recall, was always fast asleep, snuggled up in his fringed blue woollen blanket.

At the time when these existential dilemmas surfaced, my family lived on a natural gas company compound in the country, beside a paved highway which led east to Saskatchewan and west to the city of Edmonton where my numerous aunts, uncles and cousins lived. From my window I could see the dirt track on which I biked to school and which crossed the highway at the foot of Gallanger's Hill. This lane was bordered by wild rose bushes and the Reghier family farm. My brother and I were good friends with Arthur, the youngest of the thirteen Reghier children, many of whom had already grown up, moved away and started families of their own. The farm was located about a mile or so from the small prairie town of Tofield, Alberta. Being summer, the sun was high in the sky, the birds in full song.

Why then was I stuck inside with nothing to do except wonder WHY?

Why was I not outside, playing with Arthur and his nephew, who was only two years younger than his Uncle Arthur?

Why were we not swinging in the hay loft?

Why were we not draped over the wooden boards of the sow's pen watching her suckle her piglets?

Had I been born in India my questions of who, why, where and when, would possibly never have come up. And not because the summer sun sets earlier and more quickly in India, but more likely because I would have already been told by my family that I was exactly who I was meant to be, based on the effect of my *karma* which I had built up during my previous incarnations, and which had caused me to be who I was.

Possibly.

One of the seminal and delightful revelations that French anthropologist Claude Levi-Strauss is credited with by E. Leach in his article "Levi-Strauss in the Garden of Eden," is Levi-Strauss's claim that what gives language meaning is the mythology of the culture in which the language exists. For example, it is possible to translate the expression "Go to hell" into French, German, Italian, Spanish, Russian, Greek, Lebanese and so forth because these languages and cultures all share a Christian mythology and, therefore, know what the word "hell" means. On the other hand, if a person were to attempt to translate the myth of the Garden of Eden into Swahili, for example, the task becomes impossible. There is no word for "apple." The closest approximation might be "orange" and we all know the problems that occur when we try to equate apples and oranges. Meanwhile Adam and Eve would immediately be perceived as being brother and sister. According to Swahili mythology the first human beings were a brother and a sister.

So then, in order to rid ourselves of a little of our ethnocentricity and in order to foster a climate of mutual understanding, let us travel back in time and recap some of the events recounted in the great Indian epic, *The Mahabharata*, the wonderful mythic tale of the Bharata dynasty. The epic recounts the story of the horrific war between the Kauravas and the Pandavas, two prominent ancient royal families. It is the longest poem in world literature, containing stories within stories within stories within stories. The epic explains how all Indians came to be the sons and daughters of King Bharata, which is why India has traditionally been called Bharatam by the Indians themselves.

The most beloved part of the epic is the *Bhagavad*

Gita, the Song of the Blessed One, which is recounted in the epic at the dramatic moment before the major battle is about to begin. Surveying the armies stretched out before him, Arjuna, one of the Pandava brothers, has second thoughts. Speaking to his charioteer, Krishna, he expresses his remorse as he faces family and friends in the opposing army. The thought of killing his kinsmen—fathers, grandfathers, uncles, brothers, sons, grandsons—as well as comrades, teachers and friends overcomes him with despair and compassion. At the sight of all these people assembled nearby, all eager for the fight, he says to Krishna:

> *My limbs sink down,*
> *And my mouth becomes parched,*
> *And there is trembling in my body,*
> *And my hair stands on end.*
>
> *(The bow) Gandiva falls from my hand,*
> *And my skin, too, is burning,*
> *And I cannot stand still,*
> *And my mind seems to wander.*
>
> *And I see portents*
> *That are adverse, Kesava (Krishna);*
> *And I see no welfare*
> *Having slain my kinsfolk in battle.*

(Verses taken from Franklin Edgerton's translation of *The Bhagavad Gita* [1944])

Arjuna confesses to Krishna that he has no wish to kill anyone, even though not doing so would cost him his own life. Even if he were offered the rulership of the entire universe, he would not fight in the upcoming battle. Why then should he do so when the prize is merely the rulership of the earth?

What Arjuna does not know is is that Krishna is not simply his friend and charioteer. In reality, he is the Ultimate God, the Blessed One, who has, for the time being, adopted human form. The *Gita* recites the encounter in which Krishna explains that not fighting would be an even worse choice for Arjuna since Arjuna is a warrior. Warriors fight. That is their *dharma*. That is their duty. And the entire universe runs according to the sacred law of *dharma*.

If each person rejected their own duty, their *sva dharma*, the consequences of this action would be catastrophic. This rejection would have immediate cosmic repercussions. Arjuna must fight. And just so Arjuna can have no second thoughts about this, Krishna appears to Arjuna in all his transcendent awful glory. Humbled and terrified Arjuna bows before his Divine Lord, picks up his bow, *Gandiva*, and joins the fray, knowing it is not for mortal man to understand the workings of the sacred magic by which God projects the universe. It is only for him to do his duty and worship the Godhead.

Arjuna's decision notwithstanding, as the *Mahabharata* vividly portrays, the outcome of the battle is so catastrophic that it initiates the commencement of the

Kali Yuga, the final stage of the current world emanation, where the sacred cow of *dharma* stands tottering on one leg only.

Duty is one of those words that I don't hear people using much these days. I suppose it is too old-fashioned for audiences conditioned by advertising to believe that they deserve to have their every wish fulfilled. Duty is a word we are most likely to hear at Remembrance Day celebrations, although bravery, sacrifice, and hero are the more likely words to be chosen.

The words we use are vitally important. Speaking and naming have ancient roots in our collective memory. Spelling and magic go hand in hand. It is not for naught that there is a big OW in VOW. Swearing sacred oaths and living up to them is what heroes and heroines do.

Times of trouble are when we are tested and prove our mettle.

"Strength does not come from winning," said Mahatma Gandhi. "Your struggles develop your strengths. When you go through hardships and decide not to surrender, that is strength."

CHAPTER FOUR

Wilderness

When I was ten years old, my father received his twenty-year service pin from Northwestern Utilities, and decided it was time he moved his family to British Columbia. The moment had come for him to change jobs and return to the province of his boyhood, especially since the fishing was so much better there.

In 1957 the community of Prince George, BC was a small city, located in the centre of the province, at the confluence of the Nechako and Fraser Rivers. Forestry was the main industry, and the fish in the neighbouring streams, rivers and lakes were abundant. Fortunately for me, my parents had close friends, Rita and Harold Atkinson, who lived in a trailer at the Forest Station on McLeod Lake where Harold was the Forest Ranger. McLeod Lake was ninety miles north of Prince George and most of the road was gravel. I recall spending hours travelling on this road in the family car, ducking and holding my breath till the dust and gravel settled whenever we met oncoming traffic. Passing a logging truck was suffocating. Pock marks and cracks in the windshield, inescapable. En route to the Atkinsons the whole family was always on the lookout for moose. Being the first one to see the ungulate and shout "Moose" was my father's favourite game. On the prairies it had been being the first to spot a water tower and shout "I see the water tower, I see the water tower."

The Atkinsons did not have any children and were happy to have me come and stay with them whenever school holidays and my parents allowed. Although Harold and Rita must have enjoyed my company, I was the more thrilled to be allowed to stay with them. I loved fishing, whether it was trolling from a boat, casting from shore or fishing through the ice.

In the late 1950s, living on the northernmost shore of McLeod Lake, where the Pack River flowed out of the lake at the beginning of its long journey to the Arctic Ocean, was my first taste of living in pristine wilderness. I remember feeling awed by the thought that *I am the first person to walk here.* The feeling of being immersed in a wholly natural world, untouched by human beings, was omnipresent, but somewhat misleading. The McLeod Lake Forest Station was located directly across the lake from the McLeod Lake Reserve, on which many of the *People of the Rocks* still lived in teepees. And Fort McLeod, which explorer Simon Fraser had built in 1805 to facilitate the fur trade, still stood, even though its roof had caved in.

Two lessons stand out.

Early on I learned to keep my bearings. I was constantly warned not to get lost in the forest. If I got lost the chances were high that I would never be found, and I would die.

The second lesson was a corollary of the first. I implicitly understood that my life and wellbeing were irrevocably linked to other human beings. I understood that I owed my existence to the communities of people with whom I lived; that we all needed each other to survive.

Living in the wilderness in small communal groups has shaped our DNA. We share over ninety-eight percent of our genetic code with chimpanzees. Like them we historically lived in small, familial groups where we collectively cared for each other—including the young, the sick, the disabled and the old. Like them, we fought enemies for hunting and gathering rights. Like them we made tools, plotted to gain power and status, occasionally murdering one of our own to achieve this. Like them we loved, we lied, we laughed, we sorrowed, and we felt awe at the beauty of nature. Like them we even danced for rain.

Caring for each other and empathy are at the core of who we are. Like chimpanzees and other apes, human beings are social animals who are designed to live and co-operate in groups. In social animals a sense of fairness is innate. We work best within a manageable group of familiar faces. As hominids we have a well-honed ability to remember and recognize facial features. My children and grandchildren, for example, began to "make strange" when they were about six months old. Family members are loved; strangers feared.

Tragically, though, as James Lovelock remarks in *The Vanishing Face of Gaia*, "we are still aggressive tribal animals that will fight for land and food. Under pressure, any group of us can be as brutal as any of those we deplore: genocide by tribal mobs is as natural as breathing, however good and kind the individual members of the mob may be."

Living in the wilderness has shaped us over millions of years. In our contemporary urban, industrial, technological societies it is easy to forget this. It is especially easy to forget this as the wilderness rapidly disappears. Today seventy percent of the land mass of the Earth has been reshaped by human beings, earning our present age the name *Anthropocene*—a term created by geologists to describe Earth's most recent geologic era. Humans are now the number one factor altering Earth's atmosphere, land, waters, and biospheres. And we are continuing to do this at an ever-accelerating pace. Now we are on the brink of the largest extinction of species since the dinosaurs.

In the early years of recovery from his stroke, when Ron was still editing for Oolichan Books, the publishing company he founded in 1974 and sold in 2009, one of the manuscripts he worked on was Jon Turk's *Crocodiles and Ice: A Journey into Deep Wild*. In the central part of this book, Turk describes his three-month circumnavigation of Ellesmere Island, by kayak, with his companion, Erik Boomer, commencing in early May 2011. Near the end of their odyssey, he describes one of the many profound insights he experienced:

> Right here, watching the ice move, I felt that I was in the planetary clockworks, holding on to the big second hand and flying around in

great arcs, legs spun out by centrifugal force, gears spinning behind me. The clockworks of a planet. The ice had become an emotion. My own frailty had become an obvious and glorious emotion. This is what ... we now call Deep Ecology—a fundamental, innate empathy for the "living environment as a whole," and a tactile appreciation for the inter-connectivity of nature.

You don't have to go to the Arctic to see and feel the Earth's changing moods. Changes in the seasons, at any latitude or in any ecosystem, occur in abrupt fits and starts, less dramatic than the breakup in the Arctic icepacks—to be sure— but real and observable nonetheless. I believe that the first step in reining in our headlong rush toward human-induced climate change is to watch spring unfold and realize how quickly the Earth systems can change. Once we internalize local weather and seasonal change, as an emotion, once we love it, as family, then perhaps we can grasp the less visible change in our larger systems. And then, maybe—hopefully—we will be motivated to implement the concrete political, economic, and technological initiatives to do something about it. (p. 152)

In his book, *Desert Solitaire: A Season in the Wilderness*, based on his time spent as a Park Ranger in Arches National Park in eastern Utah in 1956 and 1957, Edward Abbey writes:

Wilderness. The word itself is music:

Wilderness, wilderness ... We scarcely know what we mean by the term, though the sound of it draws all whose nerves and emotions have not yet been irreparably stunned, deadened, numbed by the caterwauling of commerce, the sweating scramble for profit and domination ... wilderness invokes nostalgia, a justified not merely sentimental nostalgia for the lost America our forefathers knew. The word suggests the past and the unknown, the womb of earth from which we all emerged. It means something lost and something still present, something remote and at the same time intimate, something buried in our blood and nerves, something beyond us and without limit.... But the love of wilderness is ... also an expression of loyalty to the earth, the earth which bore us and sustains us, the only home we shall ever know, the only paradise we ever need ... Original sin, the true original sin, is the blind destruction for the sake of greed of this natural paradise which lies all around us— if only we were worthy of it.

Now when I write of paradise ... I mean not only apple trees and golden women but also scorpions and tarantulas and flies, rattlesnakes and Gila monsters, sandstorms, volcanoes and earthquakes, flash floods and quicksand, and yes—disease and death and the rotting of the flesh. (pp. 166–167)

Wilderness: A place where there are no security cameras.

A place where you can risk your life and find your soul.

The point I am trying to emphasize here is that we have evolved in the wilderness over millions of years as social animals who *collectively* care for themselves, their families, their clans, their tribes and the landscapes they inhabit. We have an innate sense of fairness and empathy and we know that losing our own health while caring for another is not right. Caregiver burn-out should never happen. Respite care should be a right. And, as more and more contemporary research is demonstrating, the best places to recuperate and rejuvenate are natural ones.

We need to dig in the earth.

We need to babble with brooks.

We need to walk barefoot in the grass.

We need to hug trees.

We need to bathe in a forest.

We need to spend time with healthy people, in healthy places.

Our individual and collective well-being depends on it.

CHAPTER FIVE

Matter

When James Lovelock, the British scientist who invented the electron capture detector, was invited to the Jet Propulsion Lab in California in 1961 by NASA to design instruments which could test for the existence of life on Mars, he did not expect the endeavour would cause him to re-imagine his ideas about life on Earth. The attempt to grapple with the essential characteristics of life so that it would be possible to design a test for life on Mars caused him to develop his Gaia hypothesis about our home planet, Earth.

The assumption Lovelock began with was that if Mars had no life then its atmosphere would be static, a state he termed *chemical equilibrium*. Gases in the atmosphere would not react with each other since there would be no organisms using these gases as a source of raw materials and as a place to deposit their waste. His hypothesis was confirmed by the French astronomers, Janine and Pierre Connes, whose spectroscopic data revealed that the atmospheres of Mars and Venus were primarily comprised of carbon dioxide with low levels of oxygen and nitrogen, etc. Furthermore, their atmospheres lacked any sign of chemical reactivity. Hence there would be no life on these planets.

Earth, Lovelock's control planet, was the planet he knew held life. By contrast with Mars and Venus,

Earth's atmosphere is "profoundly at disequilibrium." Not only are oxygen and methane present in large amounts, but these amounts have also remained fairly constant for the past million years, as ice core analyses have shown. This was an astonishing result, for, in the presence of sunlight methane oxidizes and, after a mere sixty-seven years, about two-thirds of this gas should have disappeared. The fact that the amount of methane had remained nearly constant implied for Lovelock a "disequilibrium with an astronomical improbability."

The extraordinary conclusion that Lovelock came to was that, for the past three billion years or so, the Earth and the organisms who live on her, have been regulating and maintaining the temperature and chemical composition of her atmosphere in order to nourish and sustain life—in the oceans and on the land. In discussing his ideas with his then neighbour, the novelist, William Golding, Golding suggested that Lovelock call his hypothesis the Gaia theory, after the Greek goddess Gaia. According to Greek mythology Gaia was the Earth goddess—the primordial goddess who emerged out of chaos to become the mother of life. According to Lovelock, in the dynamic exchange between the organic and inorganic systems on the planet, the Earth has continued to self-regulate to maintain the temperatures and conditions needed to sustain life. According to this view, it is possible to see the Earth herself, as a living, breathing organism.

If we believe Lovelock, the first caregiver was Gaia, herself.

As caregivers, when we care for and nurture life, we are following the primal impetus of our home planet, possibly the most deeply ingrained instinct of all—the drive to foster and nurture life in all its myriad, and magnificent, and mystifying forms.

I was twenty-eight years old when Ron's and my daughter, Nicole, was born, despite our conscious intentions to the contrary. In 1974 we believed that not having children was a lifestyle choice that had much to recommend it. Fortunately for us my intra-uterine device failed, and I remember remarking, a few months after Nicole was born, that living as I did in a technical, industrialized world, it was reassuring to know there was still room for the occasional miracle.

When I learned I was pregnant and my doctor, Gavin Brown, had removed the hapless IUD, I became witness to the mysterious truth that my body was completely capable of handling, ON ITS OWN, the nurturing of a zygote. My body knew (though I did not) how to guide the fertilized ovum through the trimesters of gestational development. My cells knew (though I did not) when and how to turn on and off the required genes, depending on the uterine environment, until the foetus was ready to leave the womb, and a human infant arrived—the process known as childbirth, the time when nature chews up a pregnant female, racks her total being and spits her out as BRAND NEW MOTHER.

Our planet Earth, as far as we now know, is the only one which supports life in the entire universe. When the Earth's systems are stressed, the Earth seeks to compensate and recreate balance. When one of her life forms is sick or injured, the impetus back toward health is strong. We have grown up in an age which continually celebrates the advances in medicine. Heart transplants, liver transplants, lung transplants, and so forth. But without the work of the cells of the body to heal the wounds the surgeons make, none of their miracles would be possible. Our own bodies are the true wonders. And they are part of the wonder that is life on Earth. The problem is that we aren't aware of this in our normal, waking consciousness, so we do not treasure our bodies or the microscopic organisms that support us.

From 1940 to 1954 the novelist, Malcolm Lowry, and his wife, Margerie, lived in a squatter's shack on the beach at Dollarton near Vancouver. Here Lowry wrote many books about the redemption of an autobiographic character, the alcoholic, Sigbjørn Wilderness. During these years it was Lowry's daily task to bring home their water. Each day he would walk along a forest path to a spring where he collected the water he and his wife needed in a canister. On returning home one day the sun came out while it was still raining. The beauty of the rain falling in the inlet through a pale silver light so enchanted Margerie that she was moved to describe the raindrops to Lowry as if he were as innocent as a child:

"You see, my true love, each [drop] is interlocked with other circles falling about it," she said. "Some are larger circles, expanding widely and engulfing others, some are weaker smaller circles that only seem to last a short while…. The rain itself is water from the sea, raised to heaven by the sun, transformed into clouds and falling again into the sea." (*Hear Us O Lord From Heaven Thy Dwelling Place*, 1961, p. 241)

The wonder with which his wife spoke about the "simple beauty" of the water cycle made Lowry realize that he had understood something of this cycle, but he had not known that the sea itself "was born of rain." And he also realized that the separation of human beings from the earth had become so great that children born into a city like Liverpool might never find anyone who would think to explain to them the wonder of rain falling into the sea. This being the case, Lowry asks if anyone "can be surprised that the very elements, harnessed only for the earth's ruination and man's greed, should turn against man himself?"

In 2012 Thomas King published *The Inconvenient Indian: A Curious Account of Native People in North America*. In it he gives such a graphic description of the "earth's ruination and man's greed" that I need to quote it here, because, unlike King, I think too many people are ignorant of "the facts and figures:

The Alberta Tar Sands is an excellent example of a non-Native understanding of land. It is, without question, the dirtiest, most environmentally insane energy-extraction project in North America, probably in the world, but the companies that are destroying landscapes and watersheds in Alberta continue merrily along tearing up the earth because there are billions to be made out of such corporate devastation. The public has been noticeably quiet about the matter, and neither the politicians in Alberta nor the folks in Ottawa have been willing to step in and say "Enough," because, in North American society when it comes to money there is no such thing as enough.

We all know the facts and figures. Carbon emissions from the production of one barrel of tar sands oil are eight times higher than the emissions from a conventional barrel. The production of each barrel of tar sands oil requires at least three barrels of fresh water, ninety percent of which never makes it back into the watershed. The waste water ends up in a series of enormous tailing ponds that cover some fifty square kilometres and is so poisonous that it kills on contact. It is only a matter of time before one or more of the earthen dams that hold the ponds in place collapse and the toxic sludge is dumped into the Athabasca River.

Just as disturbing are the surreal structures that have begun to appear on the Alberta landscape. Sulphur, a by-product of the bitumen-to-oil process, is being turned into large blocks and stacked in high-rise piles on the prairies because no one knows what to do with it. Predictably these blocks are slowly decomposing, allowing the sulphur to leach out and spoil the ground water.

Yet, in spite of all the scientific evidence, oil corporations, with the aid and abetment of government, are expanding their operations, breaking new ground as it were, and building thousands of miles of pipelines....

[T]here is little chance that North America will develop a functional land ethic until it finds a way to overcome its addiction to profit. Unfortunately there are no signs that that's going to happen any time soon. (pp. 219–220)

The Earth's biospheres are becoming stressed towards tipping points from which there is no return. Of this "inconvenient truth" we are updated with daily reminders, if only we had the ears to hear. It is in the nature of apes like us to tinker with the natural world, to invent tools to re-shape it according to our needs and, increasingly, for our wants. In our haste and in our greed, we are performing matricide.

We are polluting the Earth's waters—her springs, her brooks, her streams, her rivers, her lakes, and her oceans. In the process we are killing the microscopic zooplankton, the creatures at the bottom of the ocean's food chain upon which all the bigger creatures depend;

and we are killing the phytoplankton which produces the very air that we breathe through photosynthesis. Meanwhile we wage slaves (and compulsory retirement investors in stock markets) willingly engage in this wanton destruction for an economic system that never factors the costs of clean water and clean air into its balance sheets. It only cares for its bottom line while plotting its next equation: the development of Artificial Intelligence and the concomitant Robot Revolution, which could make all workers redundant. Unlike humans, robots are built to work 24/7 for nothing.

In 1898 H. G. Wells published an early science fiction novel, *The War of the Worlds*. The novel has a straightforward plot. Martians land on Horsell Common in Surrey, England, and proceed to wage war against humans—a war in which the humans are quickly defeated because of the invaders' superior weapons. Yet, within twelve short days, the invaders start dying and the Earth is miraculously saved. The heroes of the story turn out to be "putrefactive bacteria," microscopic organisms against which the extraterrestrial Martians have no inherited immunity. Humankind is saved thanks to microscopic life forms whose existence and importance it had previously been unaware.

Today the moral of the novel is still timely. In our wanton destruction of the ecosystems of our planet we risk killing the very organisms that keep us alive, of whose life we are mostly oblivious, and whose vital importance we do not understand. In our ignorance we take our planetary life-giving systems for granted. We pollute the air we breathe and the water we drink. We assume clean air and clean water are infinite. Similarly, we take caregivers for granted. We assume they are robots who can work 24/7 without pay or holidays.

What we need is a revolution. What we require is a society which reveres and nurtures life. We need to put caregivers of every description at the top of our economic pyramid instead of forcing them to the bottom. We desecrate life givers at our peril.

CHAPTER SIX

Mind

My husband, Ron, has often said to me that "only the imagined is possible." He believes this applies to everything, whether *the imagined* be the dream of a god, or a "theory of everything," or a poem, or a fantasy world in a novel, a television show or a movie. The products of our mind become realities. Thomas King agrees. As he makes abundantly clear in his 2003 Massey Lecture Series, *The Truth about Stories*, the kind of stories we tell each other matter. According to King, if we tell creation stories where co-operation and serendipity and humour combine, the type of societies we live in will reflect these stories. Wealth will be shared; co-operation valued; respect for the bounty of the world and the animals and plants who live in it, a given.

Caregiving, the norm.

When writing about the role of myth in life, anthropologist Branislaw Malinowsky demonstrated "that an intimate connection exists between the word, the mythos, the sacred tales of a tribe, on the one hand, and their ritual acts, their moral deeds, their social organization, and even their practical activities, on the other." Myth, he said, is not merely a story told. "It is a reality lived."

On the Pacific Northwest where I have been privileged to dwell for most of my adult life, there is prolific archaeological and oral evidence which testifies to the existence of human beings living here continuously for over ten thousand years. Thanks to the abundance of the marine and terrestrial environments, and to the knowledge of the indigenous peoples who lived here and who practiced a sophisticated "mariculture," which included building thousands of clam gardens (some of which are more than 3,500 years old) all along the coastline from Alaska to Oregon, healthy, adaptable, artistic cultures thrived. A population of over a million people inhabited the Fraser Valley, the Lower Mainland and the Gulf Islands alone—a small part of the whole territory.

In my study of the religions of the world I learned that, for the most part, so-called "primitive societies" told stories that placed every individual in their communities in fundamental relationships that bound them to their families, their elders, their clans, their tribes, their ancestors, to the animals and plants in their immediate environments, to the Earth and to the cosmos beyond. Everyone had their place, and everyone was important.

In the face of corporate homogenization, languages and cultures are rapidly going extinct. According to a recent UNESCO prediction there are currently 6,000 languages spoken globally. By the year 2050 the United Nations Educational Scientific Cultural Organization reckons there will be only 500. In the "Fourth World," the world where people live beyond the current industrial norm, the environments and cultures which support those languages are also going extinct. Gone are the days when an individual of a tribe was so familiar with its entire technology and culture that s/he could reproduce it on her own in the event of a dire emergency.

According to a 2018 UN Report on Climate Change human beings have only twelve years to avert runaway climate change. In its Fifth Assessment Report the IPCC (Intergovernmental Panel on Climate Change) stated that "There is alarming evidence that important tipping points, leading to irreversible changes in major ecosystems and the planetary climate system, may already have been reached or passed. Ecosystems as diverse as the Amazon rainforest and the Arctic tundra may be approaching thresholds of dramatic change through warming and drying. Mountain glaciers are in alarming retreat and the downstream effects of reduced water supply in the driest months will have repercussions that transcend generations."

This new reality is alarming for everyone. We have now truly entered The Unknown Zone. Ron and I fervently hope that our children and grandchildren will have a future to match the past that we have had. We want them to live, to love, to imagine, even though they will necessarily suffer, experience loss, and ultimately die. We want their children's children to live. We want all of them to live a full human life, to know they were "blessed on this Earth."

As a caregiver, I believe that climate change is also a pressing feminist issue. There are too many billions of people for the Earth to support, especially in the affluent lifestyle to which too many of us have become accustomed. If we want to halt population growth, one of the best things we can do is educate girls. Educated women have fewer children. Educated women become entrepreneurs, doctors, mechanics, scientists, engineers, plumbers, carpenters, bank managers, astronauts and pilots, as well as teachers and nurses and mothers. It has taken only a few generations to demonstrate this. Thanks to the vote and birth control, women are spilling into all the workplaces traditionally occupied by men and more men are staying home to raise children.

Unfortunately, one of the unexpected side effects of what I term the first wave of the women's liberation movement is the fact that, in North America, two wage earners are now required to meet the mortgage payments and pay the bills.

Another reality is that traditional women's work has never been properly valued, and still isn't, although some used to suggest that "the hand that rocks the cradle rules the world." Once I discovered I was pregnant, I made the choice to quit my job as a social worker and stay home to raise my child. What has always bothered me is that this decision excluded me from the only coin in which our realm reckons. I was no longer paid for the work I did. What I did was no longer deemed *valuable*. While I often quipped this was because the work I was doing was *invaluable* the reality of working as an *unpaid* housewife always grated. Fortunately, Ron earned enough money teaching at the post-secondary level that I had the privilege of staying home to raise our children. Unfortunately, today, doing what used to be the norm is no longer an option for most parents. The nurturing and educating of the next generation should be a top priority; universal daycare should be a right.

Another reality is that caregivers are traditionally women. While I personally know many men who have done and are doing a wonderful job caring for their disabled partners, it is women who are bearing the brunt of caring for the disabled, the sick and the elderly in their own families. They do this without pay or without respite care. Furthermore, the inequities in government assistance are ludicrous. Even in the province of Quebec, which does have a Minister responsible for caregiving, serious inequities still need to be addressed. For example, a single mother who is unable to work because of the 24/7 needs of her disabled child gets no government assistance for doing this. If she were to give up her child and put him into "care" foster parents would be paid in the region of $2,000 per month to do what she must do for free.

Perhaps a parallel needs to be made here. We have taken the Earth and the life she nurtures and sustains AGAINST ALL ODDS for granted. And we have taken the women who nurture and sustain the lives of their family members for granted. Perhaps it is time to remember that "Hell hath no fury like a woman scorned." When it comes to the Earth, we are just beginning to feel her wrath.

* * * * *

Societal inequities abound everywhere, not just in the treatment of women. In the space of forty years obtaining a university degree has gone from being a guarantee of obtaining well-paid employment to being, for too many, a sentence of lifelong debt.

The poor and the mentally disabled have become homeless.

The sight of little children foraging in garbage dumps is an offense against nature and humanity.

A polluted environment equals a polluted human society.

A polluted planet is a sick planet.

Like mortal human beings, whose systems all begin to deteriorate in sickness and old age, the Earth's biospheres are now all similarly compromised.

It is time for all of us to become caregivers, caregivers of the Earth and each other.

We need to imagine a better world.

We need to tell stories which celebrate the heroes and heroines who fight to achieve this.

And it is time we remembered that "Enough is great riches."

One of the things that impressed me as Ron and I travelled about speaking to stroke recovery groups, health practitioners, and general readers, was how strong and resilient people can be in the face of severe affliction.

The will to live is strong.
The brain is a marvellous organ.
Healing is always possible.

In his book, *The Wolf*, Nate Blakeshe describes what happened when wolves, which had been hunted to near extinction, were re-introduced into Yellowstone National Park. Elk numbers immediately declined, but their behaviour changed as well. They spent more time worrying about wolves and less time browsing on the willow trees by the streams. Consequently, there was more willow for the beavers to eat. Beaver populations increased.

Coyotes, however, did not fare so well. Wolves immediately cut coyote numbers in half. Rodent populations instantly rebounded. More rodents meant more food for raptors like owls and hawks. Healthier birds had larger, healthier broods. There was an "avian renaissance." Biologists who flocked to the park to study these various changes called the park's return to a state of healthy biodiversity a "trophic cascade."

What we need NOW is greater and greater areas of the Earth, from the sea beds to the mountain tops, protected in vast wilderness preserves. We need trophic cascades everywhere. We need to allow Gaia the space she needs to heal herself. And we need societies whose primary goal is the nurture and support of the people who make up them.

Let us imagine a world in which the Earth is revered, and caregivers are honoured.

Imagine full recovery. Imagine full recovery. Imagine full recovery.

CHAPTER SEVEN
Soul

When my maternal grandfather, Iver Wick, was approaching ninety years of age, he said to me, "If I have a soul, it has been a silent companion." At this time my grandfather lived on Robson Street in Vancouver. He rented a single room on the first floor of a rooming house. He had a window overlooking the street; he cooked on a two-burner electric hot plate; and shared a bathroom down the hall. The main attraction of the location was its proximity to the Vancouver Public Library, which was then situated at the intersection of Robson and Burrard Streets. Having immigrated to North America from Norway as a young man, Iver's second language was English. He faithfully read the daily newspaper, the *Vancouver Sun*, wrote numerous letters to the editor signed "The Old Shepherd," and regularly studied his *Webster's New World Dictionary*. I still have this dictionary. It's full of his marks in pencil or pen, in black or blue ink, beside those words which caught his especial attention. There is no mark beside the word *soul*. In fact, the only words which have his single vertical line beside them on the *soul* page are *sororicide*, the act of killing one's own sister, and *sorority*, a group of women or girls joined by common interests.

Like duty, soul is another word I don't hear much these days, except in relation to Black culture in the

United States, as in soul music or soul food. In my grandfather's dictionary soul is defined as

> (sōl) n. (M.E. *soule, sawle*; AS *sawol*; akin to G. *seele*, Goth. *saiwala*; only in Gmc. languages) 1. an entity which is regarded as being the immortal or spiritual part of the person and, though having no physical or material reality, is credited with the functions of thinking and willing, and hence determining all behaviour ... 4. the vital or essential part, quality or principle.

I also consulted *Webster's Encyclopedic Unabridged Dictionary of the English Language*, *Webster's New Collegiate Dictionary* and *Funk & Wagnalls New College Standard Dictionary*, and the consensus I gathered is that *soul* is separate from the body, yet it is identical with the vital or life-giving part of it. The soul departs when the body dies. Soul is akin to the Latin *anima* meaning breath, spirit, life. It is identified with many of our highest human values—nobility, warmth of feeling, spirit, courage, high-mindedness.

Soul, it seems, goes to the heart of the matter.

One of the words which was formerly used to characterize so-called primitive religions was *animism*—the belief that everything in nature had a soul. Trees, rocks, lakes, rivers, mountains, animals, plants, insects, fish— in sum everything was animated.

I am concerned that in today's materialistic society political rhetoric seems mostly dominated by economic concerns. Saving jobs, jobs, jobs, seems to be the justification for every decision, even though the corporate provider of those jobs is only concerned with cutting costs and increasing profits. At a time when corporations are global and transcend the reach of national governments, at a time when the goal of corporate production seems to be built-in obsolescence, so that the masses will have to buy more and more refrigerators that when discarded produce more and more garbage, to cite a single example, it seems logical to me that it is only a matter of time before the societies and human beings who encourage this insanity become obsolete themselves.

I am worried we have lost our soul.

Collectively we have come to a pivotal moment in human history. Some have suggested we are at a "hinge moment" in which we are now conducting a huge, uncontrolled experiment on the Earth's capability to sustain us. We have arrived at the moment when air pollution is now the fourth leading cause of death in humans worldwide. We are even experimenting with our children's minds. In the wake of so-called technological advancement our children's learning is more and more based on screen time. When this happens, researchers have found that the children's capacities for critical thinking and empathy decline. Neuroscientist Maryann Wolf suggests in *Reader Come Home* that as teaching moves from print to digital we are rapidly losing our ability to "read deeply" and consequently we are losing our capacity to imagine and to self-reflect.

My grandfather died in 1983 at the age of 92. Ron's and my last grandchild, Anja, was born in 2018, four generations later, by my count. Not long when compared with Earth's four and a half billion years. Or when compared to the age of the oceans which formed soon after the Earth around 4.4 billion years ago. Life emerged "shortly" after that. In 2017 fossilized micro-organisms were found in hydrotherminal vent precipitates in the Nuvvuagittuq belt in Quebec which could be as old as 4.26 billion years.

First comes water, then comes life.

The first apes to walk on two legs appeared in Africa somewhere around 15 million years ago. According to the Smithsonian, our ancestors began flaking tools around 2.6 million years ago. In Morocco, at Jebel Irhoud, the remains of the first "flat-faced" *Homo sapiens* were found. These hominids used stone flint tools that had been tempered in fire. According to the

Smithsonian, these people lived about 300,000 years ago. Then, around 40,000 to 15,000 years ago, genetics and fossils revealed *Homo sapiens* became the only surviving human species. Changes in human arts and technology accrued cumulatively hereafter, significantly with the introduction of agriculture around 7,000 years ago. Then, a mere 275 short years or so ago, the Industrial Revolution began. With the introduction of fossil fuel driven machines, human beings' transformation of the Earth's resources and ecosystems to suit their own ends began in earnest. My present concern is that change in human societies is happening so rapidly that we seem more like slaves to our technologies than masters of them. As my friend Lorraine says, "When you solve one problem you create two more."

Now is the crucial time to recover our "common sense" and ask: Do we really want international corporations, electrical engineers, artificial intelligence and self-teaching computers creating the parameters in which our lives are henceforth to be lived?

Now is the time to ask "what do we value most?" And "who are the people who perform the most valuable work?"

* * * * *

Swaraj or home rule is the term that Mohandas K. Gandhi used for the Indian independence movement he led. The novel tactic which achieved this end was passive resistance. Without taking up arms, millions of Indians refused to comply with laws imposed by the British colonial government, laws which the Indians felt to be unjust. The success of this movement is testimony to the strength of passive resistance in action, to the achievements that are possible when people take back power into their own hands.

Sva raj also means self-rule. It originates in the Indian quest for *moksha*, or liberation from the cycle of rebirth. It means being the master of one's body and mind and not its slave. When one is in control of one's self, others cannot control her or him.

Gandhi had a clear idea of what constituted the good life and he had specific ideas of how to achieve it. His philosophy stressed the importance of self-governance through individuals and through community building, where each one was self-sustaining, capable of providing for all their own needs—their own food, their own clothing, their own shelter. His ultimate goal was political decentralization. When people are masters of themselves, they have no need of political masters.

Today we do not have time to ask: What is the good life and how do we achieve it? Our imperative is more basic than that. We must ask: What fosters life and how do we encourage it? Clean air and clean water need to be our prime directives. To do this I believe we need to make some magic.

How we treat each other reflects how we treat the Earth. What each person does matters. In the words of the *I Ching* the higher elements must sacrifice to help the lower elements. Only collective moral force can unite the world. In this endeavour our thoughts can be creative material agents. Our survival as a species will be dependent upon our evolution as caregivers.

Making the connection between full-time caring for a family member or a friend and caring for our home planet, the Earth, seems to me a natural coupling to make. I consciously made it while I was outside forest bathing, imagining myself a forest dweller, raking and meditating and revelling in the wonder of the life around me.

The essence of magic, as I understand it, is that one thing can stand for another, that the part can stand for the whole. In the mystical thinking of Saint Teresa, while she was washing the feet of the beggars of Calcutta, she imagined herself to be symbolically bathing the feet of Christ. By bathing the feet of the beggars of Calcutta, by serving the poorest among us, she was imitating her Lord.

Similarly, I believe that in caring for the one we can symbolically care for the Earth. Over my years as a caregiver, I have come to see my relationship with family and friends as a microcosm of my place within society, nature, and the universe. Why should my sense of connectedness to Ron be any different from the garden I tend, the stars I observe in a night sky, or the meal I prepare for friends?

In loving the one, we can love all. The part can stand for the whole. Together we can make magic.

"Individually we are one drop, but together we are an ocean." —Ryunosuke Satoro

Some Phone Numbers for Caregivers Seeking Help

Since I live in the province of British Columbia, Canada, caregivers who live in other provinces or countries will need to check for comparable resources where they live. Hopefully the numbers that I have provided below will provide a useful guide to the services available in other places.

9-1-1

The emergency telephone number in North America for any situation that requires immediate assistance from the police, fire department or ambulance.

8-1-1

The toll-free provincial non-emergency health information and advice phone line that is available 24 hours a day 7 days a week in Alberta, BC, New Brunswick, Newfoundland, Nova Scotia, PEI, Quebec and Saskatchewan. (In BC have you or your spouse's BC CareCard or BC Services Card ready.)

7-1-1

The number for the deaf and hard of hearing.

2-1-1

The number to call for information about health, social services and seniors' programs.

Health Regions

In Canada, health is a provincial responsibility. In British Columbia the Ministry of Health has created five Health Regions:

Fraser Health Area	1-855-412-2121
Interior Health Area	250-980-1400
Island Health Area	1-888-533-2273
Northern Health Area	250-565-7317
Vancouver Coastal Health	604-263-7377

Depending upon where you live, call comparable numbers to get information about the Home and Community Care Services available in your area. You can also get the local phone numbers of the people you need to call to determine what programs and services you might qualify for.

Other Resources

- Call your local physician.
- Call Family Caregivers of BC's Caregiver Support Line, available Monday to Friday from 8:30 a.m.

to 4 p.m.: 1-877-520-3267. The Family Caregivers of BC (FCBC) also has a wonderful website: www. familycaregiversbc.ca. It is easy to navigate and full of important information about the support that is available for caregivers. I would also recommend calling the Caregiver Support Line for personalized suggestions: disease specific caregiver resources; their Senior Services Directory, etc. Sign up for their newsletter, join a support group, participate in webinars, listen to podcasts, and more.

- There is a Carers Canada group which is a network of organizations like Family Caregivers of BC with links to international groups: www.carerscanada.ca.

Works Cited

Abbey, Edward: *Desert Solitude: A Season in the Wilderness.*

Ackerman, Diane: *One Hundred Names for Love.*

Beauby, Jean Dominique: *The Diving Bell and the Butterfly.*

Blakeshe, Nate: *The Wolf.*

Campbell, Joseph: *The Hero with a Thousand Faces.*

Csikzentmihalyi, Mihaly: *Flow: The Psychology of Optimal Experience.*

Doige, Norman: *The Brain that Changes Itself.*

Edgerton, Franklin, translator: *The Bhagavad Gita.*

Geddes, Gary: *Vancouver Sun*, book review, "Riding the Wild Horse, Memory."

Hanh, Thich Nat: *The Miracle of Mindfulness.*

Hanh, Thich Nat: *No Death, No Fear.*

Hill, Michael. *Brain Attack: The Journey Back.* Volume II.

Kaku, Michio: *The Future of the Mind.*

Kennerley, Helen and Udo Kischka: *Surviving Stroke: The Story Of a Neurologist and His Family.*

King, Thomas: *The Inconvenient Indian.*

Klein, Bonnie Sherr: *Out of the Blue: One Woman's Story of Stroke, Love, and Survival.*

Lovelock, James: *The Vanishing Face of Gaia.*

Lowry, Malcom: *Hear Us O Lord from Heaven Thy Dwelling Place.*

McCrum, Robert: *My Year Off: Rediscovering Life after a Stroke.*

Milne, A.A.: *Winnie the Pooh.*

Smith, Ron: *The Defiant Mind: Living Inside a Stroke.*

Taylor, Jill Bolte: *My Stroke of Insight.*

Travland, David & Rhonda: *The Tough and Tender Caregiver: A Handbook for The Well Spouse.*

Turk, Jon: *Crocodiles and Ice.*

Wolf, Maryann: *Reader Come Home.*

Acknowledgements

Ron and I have been fortunate to live close to Nanoose Bay for most of our adult lives. When, out of the blue, Ron's brain attack struck, we had family and friends close at hand, and convenient access to medical and therapeutic resources. When life goes sideways, many are not so lucky. I have already spoken about the importance of a supportive family, a network of friends and a community close by. Most of the people I acknowledge here have already appeared in the pages of this book. All who do have my gratitude.

First, I would like to thank the doctors, nurses, therapists and staff at the Nanaimo Regional General Hospital, who saved Ron's life and helped him begin the long process of self-recovery. Special thanks to his Outpatient Rehab Team.

Thanks to Linda Ferron for listening and inviting us to participate in the first provincial Stroke Collaborative and for encouraging both Ron and I to write our books. To Pam Ramsay and Katie White who invited us to participate in the final Stroke Collaborative at which Ron read to health care practitioners from all over British Columbia. They returned home inspired by all four Collaboratives to implement "best practices" in stroke care in their local Health Regions.

Thanks to Lisa Watson for her healing massage therapy and for convincing Ron to head to a swimming pool asap. To Scott de Burca whose personal training sessions, sharp sense of humour and delightful Irish brogue ("one, two, tree ...") made the sessions fun as well as restorative. To the staff at the Fairwinds Wellness Centre who are always welcoming and accommodating. Thanks to Kathleen Falvai and the Oceanside Stroke Recovery Society for providing Ron and I with a safe harbour from which to get our bearings.

Thanks to Bev Coolican and her book club for convincing me to write this book. Thanks to David Stover of Rock's Mills Press for agreeing to publish it. Thanks to Ian and Virginia Garrioch for helping and sharing throughout the last fifty years. To Bill and Peggy New for their boundless enthusiasm for books and entertainments of all kinds. Thanks to the rest of our friends, neighbours and family. You know who you are. We couldn't manage without you.

I would like to thank Donna Hastings of the Heart and Stroke Foundation of Canada. The funding which the Foundation provides supports innovative research which continues to save and improve lives.

And thank you to caregivers of all ilks and stripes who daily assume their burdens in support of life and whose vital importance the Covid pandemic has made abundantly clear.

Finally to Ron, friend, lover and companion, whose bloody minded determination to heal carries us all forward.